Psychiatry and the Human Condition

Bruce Charlton MD
Department of Psychology
University of Newcastle-upon-Tyne

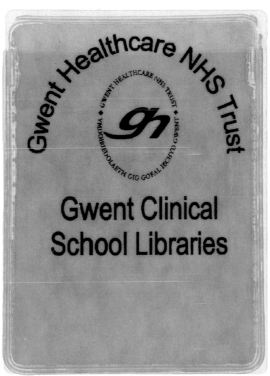

Radcliffe Medical Press

Radcliffe Medical Press Ltd
18 Marcham Road, Abingdon, Oxon OX14 1AA

British Library Cataloguing in Publication Data

A catalogue record for this book is available from the British Library.

ISBN 1 85775 314 3

Typeset by Acorn Bookwork, Salisbury, Wiltshire
Printed and bound by TJ International Ltd, Padstow, Cornwall

Contents

Preface

Psychiatric signs and symptoms – such as anxiety, insomnia, malaise, fatigue and impaired concentration – are part of life for most people, for much of the time. This is the human condition.

Psychiatry has the potential to help, and psychiatric drugs in particular have the potential to enhance human happiness and fulfilment. But there are fundamental deficiencies in the theoretical framework that guides current psychiatric research and practice.

Current classification and treatment derive from distinctions made by Emil Kraepelin some 100 years ago without the benefit of modern medicine and science. Consequently, categories such as schizophrenia and major depressive disorder now represent cultural fossils, the equivalent of obsolete diagnoses such as 'dropsy' or 'ague'. New scientific knowledge has merely been fitted around this incoherent framework. Despite consuming billions of dollars, psychiatric research has made no significant contribution to the rest of biology.

In *Psychiatry and the Human Condition*, recent research is brought to bear on the problems of classification and treatment. At present a patient would be categorised as suffering from one of the 'neo-Kraepelinian' syndromal diseases, e.g. schizophrenia or major depressive disorder. Such a patient would then be treated with a class of drug matched with that diagnosis, e.g. an 'antipsychotic' neuroleptic for schizophrenia or an 'antidepressant' for depression. The problem is that these diagnostic and drug categories are both arbitrary.

We can do better. Psychiatrists should concentrate on treating biologically valid symptoms and signs that dominate the clinical picture for each specific person. Drug choice and dosage are chosen to optimise well-being by balancing desirable against undesirable drug effects. Typically, compulsion should neither be required, nor would it be justified. If the agent and dose are tailored to individual response, most people will want to take an effective treatment – for the simple reason that it makes them feel better.

The scientific deficiencies of contemporary psychiatry are pervasive but tedious to enumerate. In this book, I have taken a positive approach by attempting to enthuse the reader with an inspiring vision of a superior alternative. The best incentive to abandon current ways of thinking and practice is the offer of something better – or, at least, potentially better.

My strategy has been to expound, as clearly and coherently as possible, a new and more rigorous way of conceptualising psychiatry. My hope is that the explanatory power of these ideas will stimulate the reader to test them in practice.

Bruce Charlton
April 2000

About the author

Bruce Charlton graduated in 1982 with honours in medicine from the Newcastle Medical School, England, and has spent much of his adult life in and around that university and city. Following a student elective at Harvard, and two Newcastle jobs as a junior psychiatrist, he went into full-time research as a Wellcome Fellow in Disorders of Mental Health at the MRC Neuroendocrinology Unit, where he completed an MD thesis on hormonal and brain changes in depression.

An idyllic interlude followed, during which he stepped outside of science and was a resident don in University College, Durham, writing an English Literature MA on the Scottish author, Alasdair Gray. After returning to medical research, he worked as a Senior Demonstrator in Physiology, a lecturer in Anatomy at Glasgow University (gaining a reference to his work in *Gray's Anatomy*), and a lecturer in Epidemiology and Public Health.

Currently, Dr Charlton is a lecturer in psychology at Newcastle University where he teaches psychiatry and evolutionary psychology, and also participates in weekly psychiatric ward rounds. He is a Visiting Professor at the UEL Centre for Health Services Research, St Bartholomew's Hospital, and a Visiting Distinguished Millennial Fellow at King's College, London.

Dr Charlton has published more than 100 papers on scientific, medical and many other topics, co-authored a book on medical education, contributed journalism to dozens of magazines and newspapers, and written a BBC Radio 3 experimental drama. He is married to Gillian Rye, who is a GP. They have a son called Billy, and live in Jesmond.

Author's note

The main argument of this book is presented such that the volume can be read straight through. I have also attempted to make the chapters *relatively* autonomous, by allowing a small degree of explanatory repetition, such that each topic could be read in any order. Further reading and references are listed at the end of the volume, and this section also presents the intellectual background to the ideas. Appendix 1 contains technical theoretical material which may be omitted, but which is necessary for a full understanding of the main argument, and ideally should be read before commencing Chapter 3. Appendix 2 concludes the book in what I hope is an optimistic spirit, by considering some of the most positive aspects of the human condition. It adopts a similar evolutionary and cognitive neuroscience-based approach to that used in the main argument of the book, but this chapter is a more easygoing meditation on the topics of ecstasy and creativity.

Acknowledgements

There are two individuals who require primary acknowledgment as the intellectual fathers of this book, namely David Healy and Antonio R Damasio. This book attempts to synthesise the conceptual breakthroughs of Healy and Damasio and to place them within an evolutionary context.

Since reading his first book, *The Suspended Revolution*, I have become ever more convinced that David Healy is the most insightful and original British Isles (he is Irish) psychiatrist of recent decades. His knowledge of phenomenology, psychopharmacology and the history of medical science is unparalleled, and exactly what is required at the present time. Suffice to say that it was Healy's work which stimulated my own return to psychiatry as the focus of my work.

David Healy has become a friend, but I have never met Antonio Damasio. However, my reading of his 1994 volume, *Descartes' Error*, was a watershed. Damasio has brought emotions within the perspective of cognitive neuroscience, and has 'solved' the ancient problem of the nature of consciousness through his discovery and explication of the somatic marker mechanism.

There are many other colleagues who richly deserve acknowledgement, and this is provided largely by means of the citations and references which follow. However, special mention should be given to Jonathan Rees and to my brother Fraser Charlton whose weekly conversations – on and around medicine and science (Jonathan), and on and around everything *but* medicine and science (Fraser) – have been a major source of intellectual stimulus over the past years.

Drs Alan Kerr and Desmond Dunleavy are consultant

psychiatrists with whom I worked in the early 1980s, and who have since made me welcome on their ward rounds. Without the timely stimulus of clinical experience which they made possible, the ideas that form this book would not have gelled.

Solitary contemplation, reading and conversation are the life-blood of my academic life as a theoretician – and the coffee-room conversation in my current Department of Psychology is particularly good. Professor Malcolm Young not only provided the niche necessary for writing this book, but was a source of vital insights concerning brain organisation and function. He has also subjected me to steady encouragement (and pressure) to get down to writing it, and has reacted with enthusiasm to ideas and enquiries. Much of the actual writing was done in the Literary and Philosophical Society in Newcastle. My editor at Radcliffe Medical Press, Gillian Nineham, commissioned this book with an excitement, swiftness and confidence that I found immensely heartening and provided important suggestions for reorganisation.

Considerable support was needed for me to complete even a slender book, as I am more naturally a sprinter than a long-distance runner when it comes to writing. So special thanks must go to Gill Rye, my wife as well as my major sub-editor, sounding board and pragmatic critic.

The understanding of nature has as its goal the understanding of human nature, and of the human condition within nature.

Jacob Bronowski

CHAPTER ONE

Psychiatry and the human condition

The endemic nature of psychiatric illness

Imagine a world in which many people suffer from psychiatric symptoms for most of the time and very few live out their lifespan without suffering periods of significant psychiatric illness. I am describing the world in which we live.

If this idea seems far fetched, try adding up the numbers. In the first place, there are the obvious individuals who suffer from the formally diagnosed psychiatric diseases such as major depressive disorder, schizophrenia or Alzheimer's dementia.

There is also the vast army of the anxious – people who go through life in a state of gnawing angst, perhaps seeking temporary relief from alcohol, perhaps stoically enduring.

Then there are those who suffer from sleep deprivation for any of a multitude of reasons – shift work, overwork, jet lag, young children, obstructed airways – or who are just chronically poor sleepers for no known reason. In addition, there are the more or less miserable people who are ill and in pain with colds, flu, hay fever, gastroenteritis, irritable bowel syndrome, headache, back-aches or inflammation. There are also the patients with life-threatening diseases such as cancers, heart disease, stroke or AIDS – who often have significant 'psychiatric' symptoms that may amount to a formal psychiatric diagnosis.

Of course, huge numbers of people at any one time will be

either intoxicated and brain impaired by alcohol, opiates, 'uppers', 'downers', solvents and the like, or else are 'hungover' and brain impaired as an after-effect of such intoxication. It must not be forgotten that prescribed drugs often have undesirable and sometimes unavoidable side-effects of a psychiatric nature, such as sedation, headaches, mental clouding, and so on. Then there are individuals without a psychiatric diagnosis but who take prescribed psychoactive medication such as tranquillizers, antidepressants, etc. These represent only a proportion of those whose state of mental health or well-being depends upon taking drugs.

When considered in this way, it is clear that few people are free of psychiatric symptoms for sustained periods of time. And if psychiatric symptoms are a matter of everyday life, then so – potentially – is their treatment. Such is the scale of the problem that professional management is inconceivable, as well as being undesirable. Logistically, this means an expansion in psychiatric self-help, which entails expertise in self-diagnosis, self-treatment and the self-evaluation of this process.

The human condition as we experience it in contemporary life is one in which psychiatric symptoms are endemic, being constantly present in the population, and also present at a remarkably high prevalence.

Disease as the norm? An evolutionary perspective

There is little doubt that, conceived in this way, psychiatric impairment is the norm. Mental health and well-being are so rare as to be remarkable. For most people, even a single day of unalloyed well-being is a rare event. Some unfortunate individuals probably never experience even a day of well-being, at best managing a few minutes as a kind of glimmering vision of what is possible.

But why should this be? Why should the world be a place of illness and drugs? Surely that is unnatural? The answer is that the modern world is indeed unnatural and has been so, for the majority of humankind, for many thousands of years. Unnaturalness is profound, inevitable and unavoidable. It is time we recognised that 'naturalness' is not an option, and worked hard on addressing how best to cope with this situation.

People are not biologically designed to be happy as such. From an evolutionary perspective, happiness is an incentive for action, not a steady state of being – it is a means to the end of reproduction. This is fundamentally why it is so difficult to achieve happiness, and why – having attained happiness – it is virtually impossible to maintain.

Humans are living in a world very different from that which shaped their bodies and minds during their evolutionary history. Ultimately, health is based upon biology, and this applies to humans just as much as to any other biological entity. Our destiny as individuals is shaped by biology. We have not transcended our dependence upon our bodies, and our minds – with their motivations, satisfactions and pains – are rooted in our bodies.

Humans are animals, and like all animals they evolved, and the circumstances under which they did so shaped their minds and bodies. The evolution of complex adaptations typically requires an accumulation of several co-ordinated genetic mutations, is gradual, and takes place over hundreds or thousands of generations. Since humans take many years to reach sexual maturity and also reproduce infrequently, the evolution of new mental capacity will have required selection pressures that were stable and sustained over time scales measurable in tens of thousands of years.

It was the ecological and social conditions of the human *prehistoric* past that shaped the minds and bodies of modern humans. Our minds were 'made up' before the invention of agriculture, and there has been insufficient time for natural selection to change them. And the evolutionary past was one in which human society was small scale, face to face, nomadic and based upon foraging, hunting and gathering.

Three types of society

For reasons which are accidental – in the sense that they were historically contingent and might easily never have happened – humans have created a range of agricultural and industrial societies with conditions that differ profoundly from the conditions under which people evolved. Natural selection is not fast enough to keep pace with the historical rate of cultural change. All across the planet, humans are dwelling in environments that, although created by humans, have aspects that are fundamentally at odds with the biological attributes with which humans have been equipped by natural selection.

The Golden Age for humans, such as it was, was the life of a nomadic hunter-gatherer. Evidence for this statement is scarce, but what evidence there is (see below) is consistent and unambiguous. This was the time when more people were happier for more of the time than at any other point in human history. It seems probable that 'modern' humans (*Homo sapiens sapiens*), our hominoid ancestors, and also the great ape human ancestors (including those similar to modern chimpanzees) lived for the great majority of their history as nomadic foragers with various combinations of gathering vegetables and hunting meat. Indeed, foraging was ubiquitous until some societies adopted village life as 'sedentary' hunter-gatherers or agriculturalists – from around 15 000 years ago.

The agrarian way of life – a life based on agriculture, herding and storage of hunted food – gradually spread to cover the whole planet. Agrarian cultures spread not because the people were happier or healthier, but by a combination of military conquest and conquest by disease. The same land could support a much larger population, with specialisation of labour to enhance productivity, and concentration of people and proximity of animals led to diseases that would almost wipe out naïve populations.

Over the past few centuries the agrarian way of life has been replaced by increasingly industrial and mercantile forms of organisation. In other words, contemporary

'Western'-type societies are dominated by production and exchange, rather than by agriculture.

Thus there are three essential types of society – nomadic foraging societies, agrarian societies (which include herding and hunting societies that use storage of food) and industrial-mercantile societies. Gellner has described the political characteristics of each of these three basic types. Essentially, nomadic-foraging societies are anarchistic democracies, agrarian societies consist of a mass of semi-starved peasants ruled by a small minority of relatively wealthy warriors with the assistance of a priesthood that propagandises on their behalf, while industrial-mercantile societies such as our own are dominated by the controllers of the wealth-creation apparatus, namely the business and money interests.

The nomadic, foraging life

Humans evolved in a society of nomadic foragers. This constitutes most of the history of the species. Most of the humans who have ever lived were hunter-gatherers. Most importantly, there have not been enough generations since humans stopped living the life of nomadic foragers for significant psychological or physical evolution to occur (although a few adaptations have evolved, such as the ability of adults to digest agricultural products such as milk, and some types of resistance to diseases of 'civilisation' such as the sickle-cell anaemia gene which gives resistance to malaria). An understanding of the conditions of ancestral hunter-gatherer life is therefore extremely useful for understanding the biological basis of human behaviour.

Although the life of our ancestors cannot be observed directly, there are indirect routes to this knowledge. Our understanding of the ancestral hunter-gatherer life is derived from a variety of sources. Naturally, this evidence is incomplete, but a great deal can be learned by combining many sources, such as archaeological evidence from relics and remains, and the anthropological study of modern nomadic hunter-gatherers who, at least until recently, lived in places such as Africa, New Guinea and South America. Observations of the behaviour of great apes and other primates and archaeological evidence of primate ancestors have also been extremely enlightening. These are supplemented by information on the history of climate, vegetation and fauna. Psychological and neurological study of modern humans, including the identification of cross-cultural cognitive patterns, can be used to explore universal and evolved mechanisms. Furthermore, mathematical modelling can be a useful way of determining the effects of theoretical changes in genes and behaviours.

A composite sketch of the hunter-gatherer life of human ancestors can thus be constructed, bearing in mind that humans did not evolve all at once, or at one place or at one time. Ancestral society was probably composed of extended family 'bands' of some 25 to 40 members. These extended families were centred around male blood relatives, and females joined from other bands of more remote relatives, probably by adolescent girls 'marrying' into the group. The bands formed part of larger, looser alliances ('clans') of around one or two hundred more or less related members with whom individuals were exchanged with some fluidity. The largest form of human organisation was the 'tribe', consisting of perhaps one or two thousand people sharing a common language. In many instances, the tribe constituted the entirety of known humanity.

Perhaps the most surprising aspect of simple hunter-gatherer societies (as exemplified by the Kung San Bushmen, or the Hazda of Tanzania) is that they are highly leisured and affluent. They are leisured in the sense that there is plenty of time for the social activities involved in preparing and consuming food, and generally gossiping, discussing and debating, co-operating and competing socially. They are affluent in the sense that the survival tasks of hunting and gathering only take up on average about half of the day (say four hours). It is the typical peasant labourer in an agrarian society for whom almost every day is composed of grinding, round-the-clock work, and whose life merits Thomas Hobbes' phrase 'solitary, poor, nasty, brutish and short'. By contrast with the life of a peasant, that of a nomadic forager is little short of idyllic.

Most people's ideas of 'primitive' or 'tribal' life are based on agricultural or herding modes of production. In such societies there is invariably domination of the mass of people by a 'chief' (plus henchmen) who appropriate a large share of the resources. However, in an 'immediate-return' or 'simple hunter-gatherer' economy there is an extremely *egalitarian* social system, with very little in the way of wealth differentials. Food is gathered on a roughly daily basis for rapid consumption, and tools or other artefacts are made as required. There is no surplus of food or material goods, no significant storage of accumulated food or other resources, and the constraints of nomadic life mean that artefacts cannot be accumulated.

Egalitarian economics

One of the most distinctive features of foraging societies, in contrast to the human societies that currently exist, was that ancestral societies were to a high degree egalitarian and without significant or sustained differentials in resources among men of the same age. There were indeed differentials in resource allocation according to age and sex (e.g. adults ate more food than children, and men ate more food than women), but there was not a class or caste system, and society was not stratified into rich and poor people who tended to pass their condition on to their children.

This equality of outcome is achieved in immediate-return economies by a continual process of redistribution through the sharing of food on a daily basis, and through continual equalising redistribution of other goods. The sharing may be accomplished in various ways in different societies, including gambling games of chance or the continual circulation of artefacts as gifts. However, the important common feature is that sharing is enforced by a powerful egalitarian *ethos* which acts to prevent a concentration of power in few hands, and in which participants are 'vigilant' about ensuring that no one else takes more than themselves. If each individual person ensures that no one else gets more than they do, the outcome is equality.

The diet of nomadic foragers was very different from the modern idea of a 'natural' diet, and equally different from the diet of agrarian peasants. For hunter-gatherers there was no 'staple' carbohydrate such as rice, wheat, oats, yams, potatoes, maize or millet – the kind of food that provides the bulk of calories in agrarian societies. Such items would, if available, have represented only a small element of a range of dozens or hundreds of vegetable foods, mainly drawn from the categories of fruits, berries, roots, tubers and nuts. This variety, and the large area over which nomads could range, meant that food would seldom have been in short supply, and foragers would not often have experienced the severe famines and chronic malnutrition that typify agrarian societies even today. For hunter-gatherers, meat probably accounted for around half of the calories, depending upon place and season. However, hunted meat differs from that which we eat today. Wild game is stringy, fibrous, high in protein and low in saturated fats. By contrast, domesticated meat produced agriculturally is often tender and fatty, so is more palatable although it is probably less nourishing.

The hunter-gatherer diet was therefore extremely varied, abundant and much more nutritious than the diet of agrarian peasant societies. This was reflected in the health and life expectancy of foragers, who were taller, lived longer, suffered much less malnutrition or starvation and had fewer diseases than peasants. Infectious disease was rare, due to the low population densities, although chronic and low-virulence infections such as syphilis and tuberculosis were a feature. None the less, the nomadic foragers who were our ancestors were probably as tall and as long-lived as almost anyone in human history except for the most prosperous classes of twentieth-century Western societies.

Degrees of happiness

The lifestyle of nomadic foragers involved little forward economic planning beyond the communal decisions of when and where to move camp, and the logistics of hunting and gathering. This means that most problems of life related to the social realm – especially concerning the question of competition for mates – and this lay behind the power struggles, disagreement, discussions and violence. And the primacy of *social* life in hunter-gatherer societies is what has been the decisive force in human evolutionary history. The main focus for natural selection is within-species, human-versus-human competition.

In summary, the ancestral hunter-gatherers experienced a way of life that was – in world historical terms – leisured and egalitarian, and they enjoyed a high level of health and long life expectancy. Of the three kinds of society as described by Gellner (1988), namely hunter-gatherer, agrarian and mercantile, it is probable that hunter-gatherers had the best life overall. Hunter-gatherer societies seem to be the happiest and peasant societies the most miserable, while industrial-mercantile societies such as our own lie somewhere in between.

That, at any rate, is the conclusion of anthropologist Jerome Barkow (1989), and his opinion is widely confirmed by the reports of many independent anthropologists who have experienced the alternatives of foraging, agrarian and industrial society. The 'naturalness' of nomadic foraging is also demonstrated by differences in the harshness of child-rearing practices in different types of society. Child-rearing involves varying elements of forcible training that are necessary to prepare children for their social role. Peasant societies typically employ extremely repressive forms of socialisation, extreme discipline, restriction, and the use of child labour. Industrial mercantile societies (such as our own) are much less harsh on children, but still require many unnatural behaviours (e.g. sitting in classrooms or examination halls for long periods of time without speaking or moving). However, nomadic foragers are able and willing to give their children even more freedom than the most liberal 'modern parent', and such a relaxed upbringing of unstructured interaction with peers apparently prepares the child adequately for the adult life to come.

Another line of evidence concerns patterns of voluntary migration. When industrial mercantile societies develop, they are popular with the miserable peasantry of agrarian societies, who flee the land and crowd the cities if given the chance. Not so the happier hunter-gatherers, who typically must be coerced into joining industrial life. My great-grand-parents left their lives as rural peasants and converged from hundreds of miles and several countries to work the coal-mines of Northumberland. They swapped the open sky, fields and trees for a life working underground and inhabiting dingy rows of colliery houses. Being a miner in the early twentieth century must have been grim, but apparently it was not as bad as being an agricultural labourer.

From a psychiatric perspective, there are sharp differences between ancestral societies and modern societies. In terms of their general social situation, modern humans are faced with a wide range of new problems, although we console ourselves with the thought that for the bulk of the population life is much better in an industrial mercantile society than in a warrior-dominated medieval peasantry. Nevertheless, we now live in a mass society full of strangers who we have no reason to trust as they are neither family nor friends. Although resources are vastly more abundant, they are linked to status and there are massive inequalities in their distribution.

This means that there is a much higher proportion of intractably low-status people in modern societies than in the societies in which humans evolved. As status is the most important factor in determining a man's sexual attractiveness, this is a major source of dissatisfaction. Men will devote enormous effort and take great risks in pursuit of the highest status, but for most people in delayed-return economies the odds are stacked heavily against them succeeding.

Improving human happiness?

Even if the impossible were somehow to be achieved and humans returned to the kind of egalitarian, immediate-return, foraging societies in which we spent much of our recent evolutionary history, unhappiness would still be common and intractable. Humans did not evolve to be happy – natural selection rewards reproductive success, not happiness. Happiness is, from this perspective, merely the 'carrot' which complements the 'stick' of pain – a lure to draw us onwards, to make us strive – but happiness is a reward that we can never permanently grasp or enjoy at leisure.

So much for the bad news. Happiness drives us, but it is not a permanent state. And this really *is* bad news because there is little we can do about it, short of changing human nature. The good news is that this might prove possible, at least to some extent. Just as human ingenuity has landed us in the predicament of a suboptimal modern human life, so the same ingenuity has provided a range of technologies of gratification through which we can attain a variety of surrogate satisfactions, something that will be discussed in more detail towards the end of this book.

Essentially the broad shape of society and its possibilities for happiness are the way they are for reasons that are accidental, unplanned and intractable. We inhabit a society that grants few satisfactions and offers limited possibilities of fulfilment. It is also a society in which psychiatric symptoms are endemic and a major cause of human misery. In our favour we have increasing knowledge of the causes of human misery, including an understanding of psychiatric illness, and increased power to alleviate that misery provided by the armamentarium of psychopharmacology. All of this understanding and therapeutic potential has arisen within the past few decades, and we have barely learned how to use it.

My point is that the human condition of Western man is intractable in its fundamentals, but amenable to improvement in important ways – things are worse than they might be. One aim of this book is to explore some of these means of improvement, and to do this will require an evaluation of the extent and nature of psychiatric illness.

The purpose of this book is therefore to suggest how knowledge and technology might be deployed to ameliorate the human condition. We are not talking about Utopia, but we are talking about the potential for significant and worthwhile improvements in well-being for substantial numbers of people. However, power can be used for many purposes, and potential agents for good are almost inevitably also potential agents for harm. The possibilities for benefit from psychopharmacology, although not universal, are nevertheless immense. Whether these benefits can be realised under the prevailing social conditions is a different matter altogether.

CHAPTER TWO

Social intelligence and the somatic marker mechanism

Social intelligence forms the basis of distinctively *human* thinking, and the somatic marker mechanism is the major embodiment of social intelligence.

What follows is a brief account of social intelligence and the somatic marker mechanism (SMM), which will suffice for the reader of the remainder of this book. However, the evidence and uncertainties which underpin these key concepts are set out more fully in Appendix 1. Anyone who wishes fully to understand the background to the ideas of this book, and to know their links with human consciousness and language, will need to grapple with the conceptual difficulties addressed in the Appendix.

Human intelligence is essentially an adaptation of social intelligence, and social intelligence comprises mechanisms that evolved for the primary purpose of dealing with other human beings. Most uses of human intelligence (e.g. watching football, doing science, playing chess, reading newspapers, etc.) are accidental by-products of this evolved ability to interpret social situations. The somatic marker mechanism (SMM) is the brain system which supports much of what is distinctive about human social intelligence – it is the way in which the brain uses emotions to interpret the meaning of social situations. 'Somatic' refers to the body, and emotions are actually the brain's interpretation of body states.

The somatic marker mechanism is so called because it is a brain mechanism which integrates body (i.e. somatic) states that correspond to emotional responses with the social situations that triggered those emotional responses. This means that emotions are used to *evaluate* social situations. In other words, perceptual information from within the body 'soma' is used to 'mark' sensory perceptual information from outside the body.

Social intelligence

The general nature and mechanism of consciousness – what it is, what it is for, and how it works – have now been largely established, at least in outline. The main protagonists in this major breakthrough have been Antonio Damasio and his colleagues. Consciousness is now situated firmly within a framework of mainstream biological research into cognitive neuroscience and evolutionary psychology. There is nothing weird or special about the brain that is involved – just normal parts of primate cerebral cortex which evolved because they benefited the organism's reproductive success.

Perhaps the most crucial advance towards a biological understanding of 'consciousness' was the development of the concept of *social intelligence*. This is the idea that the main problem which human ancestors faced, and the problem that most affected human ancestors' differential chances of reproductive success, was competition with *other people*. The social environment of the group was therefore of primary importance, not the physical environment in which the group lived. The rapid evolutionary growth of human brain size, and the distinctive aspects of human intelligence over the past few million years of evolutionary history, have occurred in response to selection pressures from conspecifics (members of the same species) consequent upon social living.

Because human consciousness and human language evolved recently, they are assumed to be aspects of social intelligence. This means that human consciousness and human language evolved and are adaptive specifically for the social tasks, and for those social conditions which prevailed at the time of rapid expansion of the frontal cerebral cortex. Consciousness was 'designed' by natural selection for dealing with other people.

However, consciousness and language are now used for many other non-social purposes, and in circumstances very different from those that prevailed during human evolutionary history. The myriad other functions and uses of consciousness and language are therefore *epiphenomena*. These non-social functions are accidental by-products, rather than capacities for which consciousness or language actually evolved. In other words, consciousness evolved to be an aspect of social intelligence, but is used for other things – just as the hand evolved its precise grip and manipulative ability to use tools, but the same ability enables some people to play the piano. Similarly, although consciousness and language are necessary for both organised religion and science, this is accidental, and the results are not necessarily adaptive.

Because of our evolutionary history, human consciousness confronts the world primarily as an instrument designed for social tasks. We tend to interpret the conscious world and the world of language as if they were inevitably social phenomena.

The somatic marker mechanism – what you need to know to read the rest of this book

- The somatic marker mechanism (SMM) is so called because changes in the inner environment of the 'soma' (body) are used to 'mark' perceptions and sensory information coming in from the external environment. This integration of bodily and environmental information occurs in working memory, which is probably situated in the upper outer areas of the frontal lobe of the cerebral cortex.

- Emotions are body states as they are represented in the brain. For example, when confronted with a threat to survival, an animal enacts a body state of physical arousal to prepare for action (e.g. heart beating fast, blood being diverted to the muscles, hairs standing on end, etc.). The brain continuously monitors the body and receives feedback from nerves and from chemicals in the blood. Fear is the emotional state which occurs when the brain recognises the physical state of arousal and adapts behaviour appropriately (e.g. generating fight or flight). Most large animals experience emotions.

- Although many animals experience emotions, only humans (and perhaps a few other complex social animals, such as chimpanzees) are capable of being *aware* of emotions. We become aware of our emotions when our attention is drawn to them, but by contrast a mouse can experience fear, but it cannot become aware of its own state of fear. 'Feelings' is the term used to refer to emotions of which we are aware, and we are aware of them because those emotions are represented in working memory.

- Working memory (WM) is the site of awareness, located in the prefrontal lobe of the cerebral cortex. WM functions as an integration zone of the brain, where representations from different systems converge, and where several items of thought to which we are attending can simultaneously be sustained and manipulated. When we deliberately grapple with a problem and try to think it through, this process is happening in working memory. When we are aware of something, it is in working memory. When we wish to attend to a specific stimulus, we represent it in working memory.

- The SMM is found only in humans and a few other social animals. It integrates perceptions of social situation with the emotions that occur in response to this situation (e.g. a particular person integrated with the emotions that they make us feel – fear, lust, surprise, etc.). The SMM is able to do this because both perceptions and emotions are represented in working memory.

- For instance, when a rival male provokes fear, the bodily

state of fear (emotion) links with the identity of the male rival (perception). Thus the SMM creates a representation in working memory. This emotional-perceptual representation can be stored in long-term memory, and when recalled it has the potential both to provoke recognition (of the male rival) and to evoke an emotion in the body (fear). Thinking about the male rival (even when he is not present) therefore *replays* the emotion of fear, which means that the body is stimulated to re-enact the same body state that was experienced at the time when the perception was laid down in memory.

• The somatic marker mechanism is here considered to be the basis of the 'theory-of-mind' mechanism. Theory of mind is the name often given to the ability of humans to make inferences ('theories') about the contents of other people's minds (e.g. knowing that someone else does not have the same ideas as I do, but rather that each person has knowledge and desires that are frequently different from my own).

• The somatic marker mechanism uses the emotional response to a social situation to make inferences about the dispositions, intentions and motivations of the people involved in that social situation. For instance, if a male rival induces the emotion of fear, then my inference might be that this male rival is hostile and aggressive. Whenever I think about that man I replay the emotion of fear, and I reason that he is intending to harm me. This is equivalent to my having a 'theory of mind' about the male rival, since it involves making an inference about what he is thinking.

• Because the somatic marker mechanism underpins human social intelligence, and because social intelligence underpins much that is distinctive about human thinking, the physical attributes of the SMM have implications for human behaviour.

• For example, the categories of distinctively human intelligence are seen to be social categories and emotional categories. It would be expected that these categories would underlie much of human thought, even when the subject matter is abstract.

- The fact that the SMM is located in working memory means that the conscious human world is essentially a social world, permeated with social categories and orientated towards social matters. Human beings see the world through social lenses.

CHAPTER THREE

Psychiatric classification

Current diagnostic practice – pragmatism

Psychiatric illnesses and diseases are classified into a diagnostic scheme or 'nosology'. The prevailing ideas are exemplified in the USA and research communities by the regularly updated editions of the Diagnostic and Statistical Manual (DSM) of the American Psychiatric Association, and in Europe (and for more epidemiological purposes) by the International Classification of Disease (ICD).

The commonly used diagnostic scheme in clinical practice owes much to the DSM and ICD, but also continues to make other distinctions which lack 'official' sanction. Thus the systems in practice include some of the familiar (although controversial) distinctions between organic and 'functional' psychoses, between schizophrenia and the 'affective' disorders, between unipolar and bipolar (manic-depressive) affective disorders, and between psychosis and neurosis and the personality disorders.

These diagnostic systems employ a syndromal system of classification that ultimately derives from the work of the psychiatrist Emil Kraepelin about 100 years ago, and is therefore termed the 'neo-Kraepelinian' nosology. Whether or not a psychiatrist uses the formal diagnostic criteria, the neo-Kraepelinian nosology has now become ossified in the DSM and ICD manuals. Over the past few decades the mass of published commentary and research based on this nosology has created a climate of opinion to challenge which is seen as not so much mistaken as absurd.

Yet the prevailing neo-Kraepelinian nosology is a

mishmash of syndromes that have widely varying plausibility and coherence. Some diagnoses are probably indeed biologically valid – having perhaps a single cause, occurring in a single psychological functional system, or having a unified pathology (for instance, some of the anxiety disorders, such as generalised anxiety, panic and simple phobias). However, from the perspective of providing a sound basis for scientific research, especially for the core diagnoses of the 'functional psychoses', the whole thing is a terrible, misleading mess.

Categorical thinking

It might be thought that the current diagnostic schemes are supported by a wealth of scientific research. However, almost the exact opposite is the case. Despite widespread scepticism in the research literature about the validity of the current diagnostic categories, it is still the case that almost all biological research is based upon neo-Kraepelinian diagnoses, rather than neo-Kraepelinian diagnoses being based on research.

A typical research project will involve comparing a group of subjects diagnosable in a DSM or ICD category with normal controls with respect to some measurable parameter, which may for example be biochemical, hormonal or some aspect of brain imaging. The biological validity of the diagnostic categories is implicitly assumed, and all information-gathering is structured around this assumption. Whether the results mean anything at all depends entirely on the validity of the comparison groups. For example, although almost no one believes that schizophrenia is a single disease entity, a vast amount of research is funded, conducted and published on the causes, correlates and cures of 'schizophrenia' and is based upon gathering groups of 'schizophrenic' patients and comparing them with other diagnoses and controls. Conferences, journals and societies are based on the diagnosis.

This has created and sustained the illusion that current psychiatric practice is a matter of diagnosing biologically individuated diseases and treating them with specific agents. The diseases are considered in categories such as depression, mania and schizophrenia, while the treatments are seen in categories such as antidepressant, mood stabiliser and antipsychotic. This is categorical thinking – that is, diseases and drugs are put into categories whether or not those categories are valid, and whether or not the individual people and drugs fit the categories comfortably. Classifying everything creates an illusion of understanding.

However, when the neo-Kraepelinian diagnostic schema has been analysed, it has typically been found that the standard diagnostic categories have less predictive validity than a symptomatic approach. In other words, treating a patient with the diagnosis of depression is really much the same as (or worse than) treating a patient's symptoms of depression, and treating the diagnostic category of schizophrenia is really more akin to treating the symptoms of hallucinations and bizarre delusions. And the treatment of a symptom such as auditory hallucinations is the same whether the symptoms occur in schizophrenia, mania or psychotic depression.

The same applies to psychiatric drugs. In reality, the categories such as 'antidepressant' and 'antipsychotic/ neuroleptic', 'anxiolytic' and 'mood stabiliser' are neither distinct nor autonomous. Psychiatric drugs (like most other drugs) have broad and non-specific pharmacological and clinical actions. To take the example of the 'antipsychotic' chlorpromazine, this has powerful antidopamine, antihistamine and anticholinergic actions. And its clinical actions, as well as the antipsychotic control of hallucinations and delusions, also include sedation and anxiolysis, a kind of a general 'strait-jacketing' behavioural control in high doses, control of mania, antidepressant activity (especially in severe psychotic depression), antinausea and anti-emetic actions (for which it was originally licensed in the USA), and control of hay fever and hiccups. Indeed, chlorpromazine is just about the least specific drug ever invented, so to regard it primarily as representative of the class of neuroleptics or antipsychotics is particularly absurd.

A new nosology needed

The continuation of the current diagnostic system therefore has little or no scientific justification, and is only supported by the pharmacological evidence through an extraordinary habit of considering psychiatric drug activity in distinct categories. Indeed, it would probably be true to say that we know enough to know that *the current nosology is untrue*.

Certainly this holds in important respects – for instance, that schizophrenia is definitely *not* a valid biological category. The diagnostic category of schizophrenia is little if at all predictive of prognosis or specific treatment response, displays no specific psychological abnormalities, has no distinctive or characteristic physical pathology, and in general does not make sense from a biological perspective. This is hardly surprising in view of the fact that the current concept of schizophrenia is a modification of ideas that are 100 years old which has never been revised in the light of modern knowledge. How many other century-old diagnostic schemes are still regarded as valid?

The only proper justification for continuing the neo-Kraepelinian approach is that it is much better than no classification at all, and that no other system is as well validated. These are compelling pragmatic reasons, and I certainly would not advocate dropping the current nosology from clinical practice until something better comes along *and has been thoroughly researched*. However, there is no reason why a new nosology should not immediately guide *research* (as opposed to clinical practice). All rationality points to the urgent need for researchers to drop the current classification at once and set to work to try to discover something better.

That is the project I shall begin in this book, namely the search for a better nosology – a better system of disease classification that is more biologically coherent and will serve as a basis for research. I shall suggest several psychiatric diagnostic categories, based upon cognitive neuroscience informed by a perspective from evolutionary psychology. And I shall reinterpret psychiatric drugs in terms of their actions upon these psychological variables.

CHAPTER FOUR

The delusional disorders

One of the classic symptoms of 'madness' is to have false but strongly held beliefs that have a powerful effect on behaviour. Such beliefs are termed delusions – at least they are termed delusions when they are taken to be a symptom of psychiatric illness. Many people who have delusions also have other symptoms of 'madness'. For example, they may hear voices, have incoherent speech, display strange or inappropriate moods or adopt bizarre postures, and are immediately recognised by the general public as 'mad'.

However, some people with delusions are entirely 'normal' except for the false belief that they hold, and the belief itself is neither impossible nor outlandish. Any other unusual behaviours can be traced back to that false belief. For instance, a man may have the fixed, false and dominating belief that his wife is having an affair with a neighbour. This belief may be so dominating as to lead to a large programme of surveillance – spying on his wife, searching her handbag, examining her clothes, etc. Yet the same man may show no evidence of irrationality in other areas of his life, being able to function normally at work and socialising easily with acquaintances, so that only close friends and family are aware of the existence of the delusion. In such instances the delusion is said to be 'encapsulated' (i.e. sealed off from other aspects of mental life), and such individuals are said to have a delusional disorder.

Case history of a persecutory delusion – the story of Bill

Bill is an unemployed man in his early thirties, who is happily married with children. Bill's delusion began two years before the interviews. He believes that a gang of criminals think he informed on them. These men want to hurt or kill him, and will do so if they see him. As a consequence, he rarely leaves the house.

One of Bill's old friends was a shopkeeper who was burgled several times over a short period of time. Bill knew no details of the crimes. However, he coincidentally went to visit shortly after a burglary had occurred, and stood outside the shop talking for a while with his friend. On the same day the shopkeeper happened to discover the burglar's identity, and Bill believes that the shop assistant will have assumed that this information had been passed on by Bill during his conversation outside the shop. As the burglars were frequent customers at the shop, the assistant will (Bill thinks) probably have told them that Bill was the informant. Bill believes that these criminals now want revenge, and may want to kill him.

Two pieces of supposed evidence have confirmed this theory. First, Bill was waiting in a car when he saw some men pointing at him and overheard them saying 'that's him in the car'. Secondly, at about the same time Bill also began to notice that old friends seemed to be ignoring him in the street, and were behaving in a manner similar to that directed at someone known to be a 'grass'. In order to avoid meeting the burglars, Bill stays at home as much as possible. If he finds it necessary to go out, he runs between his house, the car and his destination. This has stopped him having a job and being able to take his children to school, and has led him to be referred to a psychiatrist. He was diagnosed as having 'acute paranoid disorder', prescribed antidepressants and neuroleptics, and he continues as an out-patient.

Bill's case is a true story, although names and identifying

details have been changed. Yet the striking thing about Bill was how 'normal' he was. Even on detailed interviewing he did not appear in any way 'mad'; he presented socially as a very 'down-to-earth', plain-speaking, solid working man. He showed no evidence of other psychiatric illness or of intellectual damage. If not discussing the subject of his delusions he could converse with interest and animation in a manner indistinguishable from that of other men of his age and background. His persecutory beliefs were false, and were based on what seemed to most people to be inadequate evidence, yet they were not bizarre beliefs, nor was his reaction to them difficult to understand. If Bill had been correct about being persecuted, then his interpretations and actions were perfectly understandable and reasonable in the circumstances.

Delusions and other false beliefs

Delusions are typically stated to have three major defining characteristics – first, that a delusional belief is false, secondly, that this false belief is behaviourally dominant, and thirdly, that the false belief is resistant to counter-argument. All of these characteristics are shown by delusional disorders, yet they occur in a context of generally non-pathological cognitive functioning.

Humans are extremely prone to 'false' beliefs, or at least beliefs that strike many or most other people as false. Some of these false beliefs are strongly held and dominate behaviour. It is obvious that humans are imperfect logicians operating for most of the time on incomplete information, so mistakes are inevitable. However, it is striking that although everyone would acknowledge the imperfections of human reasoning, many of these false beliefs are not susceptible to argument. For example, deeply cherished religious and political beliefs are none the less based on little or no hard evidence, vary widely, yet may dominate a person's life, and are sometimes held with unshakeable intensity. And religious and political beliefs may strike the vast majority of other people as obviously false.

What about beliefs concerning the racial supremacy of people with white skins or the racial inferiority of Jews? Such beliefs have been common in many times and places, and they are certainly strongly held, affect behaviour, and a person who holds them may not be persuadable to the contrary. Although we consider them false as well as wicked, there would seem to be no compelling evidence with which we might have confronted, say, Adolf Hitler that would have persuaded him to admit he had been wrong about the Jews. Even if Hitler may be considered an insane individual, that could not apply to all of the millions of people who agreed with him.

On reflection, we all harbour beliefs that may strike other people as false, even abhorrent, yet they could not persuade us out of them, at least not over a short time scale. Deeply felt beliefs do sometimes change over a lifetime, but not necessarily as a consequence of compelling evidence. People sometimes change their political views, convert to a new religion or to agnosticism, and in their personal lives go through several revisions of their opinion about who is the most beautiful and desirable woman or man in the world.

In other words, delusions are a part of everyday life, but all of these everyday delusions are of a particular type. They are all delusions in relation to *social intelligence*. Basically, all of these false or at least unjustifiable beliefs are based upon interpretations of the human world. Even some of the more strange beliefs people have about cosmology and metaphysics often boil down to beliefs about agency – the power and influence of powerful and influential agents – whether human or supernatural.

These everyday delusions can be interpreted alongside a formal psychiatric diagnosis known as delusional disorder. The category of delusional disorder describes a psychiatric syndrome characterised by non-bizarre, chronic and content-encapsulated false beliefs in a context of generally intact affect, speech and general behaviour. In other words, a person with delusional disorder is essentially normal except for the subject matter of their delusions, and all other abnormalities of their behaviour can be traced back to that cause.

The subject matter is variable, with persecutory, jealous, grandiose, erotomaniac and somatic subtypes. A persecutory delusion might involve a fear that one is being hunted by a hostile gang, such as the mafia. Jealous delusions involve a belief in the sexual infidelity of a partner. Grandiose delusions involve the false belief that one is of higher status than one's actual status, or perhaps that one possesses exceptional powers or skills. A person subject to erotomaniac delusions will believe that someone is in love with them when that is not the case. Somatic delusions involve false beliefs about parts of one's body – for example, that one has a large ugly nose when it is actually normal.

It will be suggested that many delusional disorders can plausibly be interpreted as 'theory-of-mind delusions' – that is, false beliefs whose formal characteristics are consequences of the theory-of-mind mechanism, and whose subject matter reflects social selection pressures that were important during human evolutionary history. This analysis will in turn throw light upon the nature of human thinking about social interactions, and will demonstrate the dependence of social judgement on emotions and feelings.

The 'theory-of-mind' mechanism (ToMM) and delusions

It is striking that the subtypes of delusional disorder represent fundamental aspects of human social functioning, being related to sexual attractiveness (erotomaniac and somatic types), sexual reproduction (morbid jealousy), status (grandiose) and personal survival (persecutory delusions).

Human social intelligence has evolved in order to understand, predict and manipulate the behaviour of other people – a task that places exceptional demands on cognitive processing. It is believed that social competition between humans provided the most important constraint on survival and reproduction under recent ancestral conditions.

Social intelligence interprets behaviour in the light of inferred *mental states*. In other words, the mechanism of social intelligence makes 'theories' of mind, which are inferences about what other people are thinking – their motivations, intentions and dispositions. These inferences concerning mental states affect the interpretation of behavioural cues. For instance, a clenched fist might be interpreted either as a threat of violence or as an encouraging gesture of support, according to whether the motivational mental state was inferred to be hostile or friendly. This evolved adaptation by which states of mind are inferred and deployed in human reasoning has been termed the 'theory-of-mind mechanism' (ToMM).

The neural mechanism for the ToMM has recently been elucidated by Antonio Damasio and his colleagues and termed the somatic marker mechanism (SMM). As described previously, in essence the SMM involves using one's own emotional reactions as indicators of another person's mental state, and then using this 'cognitive representation' of person plus mental state to perform internal modelling of behavioural consequences. For example, if the approach of a stranger induces an emotional response of fear, a combined emotional-perceptual representation of a 'fear-inducing' (or 'hostile') stranger is created in working memory. If the perceptual representation of the stranger is reactivated from memory, as well as recognition of the individual the linked emotion of fear will also be redeployed in the body and physically re-experienced. The function of the perception–emotion linkage in ToM is therefore to evaluate the significance of internally modelled social situations.

Our attitude to a social situation is profoundly affected by the emotions that occur as a consequence of that social situation. This attitude is re-evoked and re-experienced as an emotion when that social situation is recollected or anticipated. Thus the social *category* to which the original social situation was assigned becomes capable of creating a particular emotion. Every time you think of the prospect of meeting Big Al you feel fear, or every time you think of Big Alison the recollection evokes a stirring of desire...

Psychopathology of theory-of-mind delusions

Since it is argued that delusional disorders are aspects of social intelligence, and social intelligence involves the ToMM, then the structure and function of the somatic marker mechanism should be able to explain many of the clinical and phenomenological features of delusional disorder.

The suggestion is that delusional disorders are a consequence of normal, logical reasoning from false premises concerning other people's mental states. The false beliefs are based on false assumptions about motivations, intentions and dispositions, rather than being a consequence of strictly logical errors.

The assumption here is that the delusional disorders occur in a context of non-pathological, adaptive cognitive processes, including an *intact* ToMM, and that their characteristic false beliefs are an outcome of the nature of psychological mechanisms operating on a particular personality type and social circumstances. A further factor is probably that human psychological mechanisms evolved under tribal conditions but now operate in a mass social environment populated mainly by strangers performing unobserved acts – what was formerly adaptive may become pathological under modern circumstances.

Subject matter of delusional disorder

Humans are social animals, and the reproductive success of our ancestors depended crucially upon their ability to negotiate the social milieu and to compete with members of their own species. Beliefs in the social domain therefore tend to have a strong effect on behaviour (i.e. beliefs tend to be behaviourally dominant) because the social arena is crucial to human survival and reproduction.

The subject matter of delusional disorder bears a striking

resemblance to the principal categories of social interaction that have evolutionary importance and require mental state inferences. In other words, delusional disorders apparently reflect the nature of social selection pressures in an ancestral environment. For example, homicide is a major cause of premature male death (and hence failure to reproduce) under tribal conditions, and many homicides are caused by 'gangs' of males. The same phenomenon has been reported in common chimpanzees, where 'gangs' from one troop will seek and kill isolated males from another troop. Persecution by hostile alliances of unrelated males was probably a significant feature of ancestral social life, and it makes sense that inferences concerning persecution by male alliances have the potential to act as a powerful influence on behaviour.

Similarly, a conjectural evolutionary scenario to account for erotomaniac and some somatic delusions can be derived from sexual selection theory. The major variable that influences a man's attractiveness to women is status, and erotomania can be seen as a condition in which a woman becomes delusionally attracted to an unattainable but high-status male whom she believes returns her love. By contrast, a woman's attractiveness to men is primarily a matter of physical beauty (cues of youth and health), and in the *somatic* type of delusional disorder (i.e. a delusion related to the body or 'soma') a common presentation is in a hypersensitive, insecure woman of reproductive age who has become preoccupied with the notion that she is physically unattractive due to some bodily impairment (such as a foul odour) or personal ugliness (e.g. blemished skin or a large nose). Somatic delusions of this type are reported to be unusual in women beyond reproductive age. When somatic delusions of this type are found in men, it could be predicted that they will be more common among those who rely on their appearance to attract sexual partners (e.g. homosexual men, or men of lower social status).

False beliefs are unavoidable in mental state inferences

The false beliefs found in delusional disorder are social, and inevitably involve making mental state inferences (i.e. judging the dispositions, motivations and intentions of other people). Mistakes in evaluating dispositions, motivations and intentions are inevitable. Beliefs concerning the mental state of others are always *inferences* based upon insecure (emotionally derived) assumptions. They cannot *always* be true because beliefs cannot be checked against objective criteria – there is no direct access to other minds.

Inferences concerning the state and content of other minds depend upon information from one's own subjective emotional responses, as well as from observed behavioural cues. When a subjective emotional response is inappropriate, then the inference of mental state will be wrong. For example, inappropriate fear may lead to a false belief concerning the hostile intentions of a male stranger, and this may emerge as a persecutory delusion. There is no secure way of checking whether fear of another person is appropriate – whether Big Al really is as aggressive as he makes you feel he is, or whether beneath the granite exterior beats a heart of gold. The link between emotions and delusional disorder may also be seen in the reported association between low self-esteem (i.e. perceived low status) and morbid jealousy. If a man believes he is unattractive to his wife and other women, he is more likely to believe that his wife is motivated to have a sexual relationship with another man who is more attractive.

Beliefs concerning ToM inferences will be resistant to counter-argument

Beliefs concerning the state of mind of other people may be resistant to counter-argument because the human social domain is intrinsically competitive. We would be foolish always to be persuaded by the arguments of others, since everyone is 'in competition' with everyone else to a greater or lesser extent. Even close family members will lie to one another (whether 'for their own good' or to shape behaviour in a more personally advantageous direction).

Indeed, it is suggested that the ToMM evolved as a direct consequence of human-versus-human competition. We base our assessments of others on the emotions they evoke in us – 'I know everybody says he is nice, but I don't trust him – he makes me *feel* uncomfortable'. These feelings have adaptive significance. Deception and concealment of hostile motivations and damaging intentions can be expected in the social domain.

Mistrustfulness concerning the reassurances of others is, in this sense, adaptive. Dishonesty from other people – in these matters – is to be anticipated. Would your best friend really tell you if your wife was having an affair? Many people lie in such circumstances for all kinds of reasons, especially when it might be your best friend who is having the affair... It therefore makes sense that, despite their being based upon insecure inferences, beliefs concerning theory of mind will be neither labile nor readily abandoned. In a rivalrous social world where no one can be wholly trusted, each individual must reach their own conclusions about the motivations, disposition and relationships of other people.

Delusions are encapsulated due to the nature of the ToMM

When mental-state delusions are a consequence of the ToMM (i.e. the SMM), they depend on a cognitive representation that incorporates a social identity with an emotion. In other words, a body state is linked specifically with a particular category of social interaction. Thus the social category of a particular gang may be linked with the emotion of fear, and whenever the gang is thought about the body will enact the emotion of fear, and this state of fear will influence the interpretation of social events. Other social categories might include kinship categories (mother, father, spouse, son or daughter, etc.), groups in our immediate environment, or any other grouping which we (rightly or wrongly) subjectively consider to be cohesive (e.g. 'the Irish', 'the communists' or 'the managers').

However, other social categories are not linked to fear. Mental state inferences will therefore be restricted to the particular person or group described by that social category.

This potentially explains why pure cases with delusions of persecution can nevertheless maintain friendly and co-operative social relationships with people outside the social category of their presumed persecutors. Female persecutory delusions usually relate to familiar people, while male delusions relate to strangers. In both cases, the delusion is encapsulated according to social category.

The example of morbid jealousy

A jealous delusion – Edward

What follows is a true story, although the names and identifying details have been changed.

Edward is a man in his mid-twenties. He had an uneventful childhood, was an average pupil and left school – without taking examinations – to serve an apprentice-ship. Edward's personality is cautious and careful, and people have commented on his neatness, punctuality and conscientiousness. Although somewhat shy, he has plenty of friends and an active social life. Indeed, he has strong attachments to his family and a powerfully developed sense of personal responsibility. He has no history of psychiatric illness, nor current signs of psychiatric illness.

In his early twenties, Edward began a relationship with a younger girl called Frances that lasted for several years. As the relationship progressed it became more stormy, with arguments centring around Frances's desire for more freedom to go out with friends, and Edward's increasingly possessive attitude towards her and his criticisms of her sexually provocative style of dress. Edward became increasingly worried that Frances might be 'seeing other boys and having sex – if she had sex with anyone else I could never have her back'. The worry escalated into a tormenting preoccupation, and on one occasion Edward was driven to phone one of Frances's friends to check that she was not seeing anyone else. On another occasion he went around the local night clubs to check on her whereabouts.

The situation became so bad that the relationship split up (a 'trial separation'). However, Edward became even more distressed. One evening he saw Frances in a bar, talking to a group of men and dancing in what seemed to him to be a provocative manner. He left the bar ruminating on the possibility that she was seeing other men, and the thought 'jumped through' his mind that she might have had sex with them – although he pushed this thought aside. In an overwrought mood, he waited outside her home in his car to discuss their relationship. She sat beside him in the car, an argument broke out, and Francis tried to make it up by kissing Edward, but he exploded in sudden anger at her sexually provocative manner, and he strangled her to death.

Edward was immediately overwhelmed with remorse, drove for miles, and made a determined attempt at suicide. The interview took place in prison where he was awaiting trial for murder.

Jealousy in humans is a cultural universal, a complex and characteristic pattern of behaviour in response to specific cues, which serves an adaptive function concerned with paternal investment in offspring. Across the animal kingdom, jealous behaviour is found only when males contribute resources to their offspring (especially after birth), and is a response to the problem of uncertain paternity in species where females potentially mate with more than one male. Jealousy in men can be seen as an evolved 'instinct' that operates to reduce the likelihood of sexual infidelity in a partner, and to decrease the chance of misdirected investment. If a male were to tolerate sexual infidelity and continue to invest resources in a rival male's offspring, he would incur the 'double' genetic penalty of both failing to reproduce and 'wasting' resources on assisting a rival's reproduction. Humans have few offspring, each of which requires a substantial investment of resources. Thus any child sired by another man represents the loss of a substantial proportion of expected reproductive capacity.

Jealousy in women is significantly different in its motivation and intentions, as female mammals do not suffer from uncertainty about the identity of their offspring, and sexual infidelity *per se* is not a problem. The problem for a female is to secure investment to help in rearing offspring, and jealousy is primarily concerned with ensuring that the male partner directs his investment efforts towards the woman's own offspring. Therefore female jealousy is less concerned with the *act* of sexual infidelity and more with the danger of a male partner transferring his affections (and resources) to another female. Hence selection pressures have led to different cues that stimulate the emotion of jealousy in men and women. Men primarily fear *physical* infidelity (the partner having sexual intercourse with another man), while women primarily fear *emotional* infidelity (the partner falling in love with another woman).

'Morbid jealousy syndrome' describes a condition of inappropriate or excessive jealousy, specific to the sexual partner, and which dominates behaviour. This becomes delusional when it involves a false belief in the sexual infidelity of the spouse or sexual partner. Morbid jealousy can occur in a pure form (i.e. without the presence of another psychiatric diagnosis) in both males and females, although it is commoner in males. The extreme of morbid jealousy itself would not usually be considered adaptive, as it could severely damage reproductive success – for example, when it causes the breakup of a relationship, or death of one or both partners by homicide. However, it remains possible that the threat or possibility of such extreme sanctions may serve as an effective deterrent. Thus even intense jealousy may be adaptive on average or under ancestral conditions.

Delusions of sexual infidelity can be regarded as consequences of the ToMM and strategic social intelligence, since they are concerned with *internally modelled* social relationships and mental state inferences. Jealous delusions are not about what is happening here and now (since that is a matter for direct observation), but instead about what did happen, is happening elsewhere, or might happen in the future. False-positive or inappropriate jealousy is inevitable at a certain frequency, as imaginative construction of possible scenarios cannot always be based upon or checked against reality. Moreover, inferences concerning the intentions of a sexual partner are not directly accessible but can only be checked against behaviours whose interpretation is ambiguous.

Jealousy is notoriously resistant to reassurance or counter-argument. There is often no objectively convincing way in which to contradict the delusional belief. This arises from the fact that jealousy evolved in a context of social competition where deception is expected as an element of that competition. None the less, false beliefs of sexual infidelity are compatible with being encapsulated and specific to the sexual partner. The encapsulation occurs on the basis that the ToMM involves a cognitive linkage between a particular social category and the particular emotions associated with jealousy. Outside that subject matter and that emotion, cognitive life may continue relatively unaffected.

Thus the emotion of jealousy may be 'attached' to the social category of 'my wife' and confined to that category. A man who is jealous of his wife need not be jealous of any other woman ('he always seemed charming to me. . .'), or of women in general, or of men, or of inanimate objects. Sexual jealousy is probably always confined by category, although the category will vary between individuals and may be more extensive than, for example, just wife (e.g. sexual jealousy may apply to any women with whom the man has had sexual relations, or any woman with whom he wishes to have sexual relations). The point is that, due to the SMM, the emotion is linked to a perceptual category such that evocation of the perceptual category triggers the emotion.

Patients with delusions show varying degrees of rational 'insight' into the possibility of error in their inference, and

ToM delusions, including non-delusional morbid jealousy, may respond to reasoning techniques such as cognitive-behavioural therapy. However, a fundamental problem for cognitive therapy of delusional disorders concerns the intractable inaccessibility of the true intentions and motivations of others. It may be impossible in practice to prove a negative – for example, that a partner has *not* been sexually unfaithful or that there is *no* gang trying to kill you, or that *secretly* men find you repulsive and stare at your big nose, or for that matter that Big Alison finds you almost overwhelmingly attractive and has to fight very hard to avoid showing the fact. . . .

Theory-of-mind delusions are part of 'normal' life

In these ToM delusions relating to social instincts, the delusional quality (i.e. its dominating and intractable nature) is a consequence of the evolutionary importance of the subject matter combined with the frequently insurmountable difficulty of verifying mentalistic inferences. The intensity of a false belief may wax and wane quantitatively between morbid preoccupation and frank delusion according to personality and social circumstances, and will typically persist in the long term. It follows that the exact dividing line between a ToM delusion and a strongly held and dominating 'overvalued idea' is of little pathological or diagnostic significance.

The suggestion is that delusional disorder is understandable in terms of evolved psychological mechanisms for making mental state inferences. 'Theory-of-mind delusions' are an inevitable consequence of the ToM depending upon subjective emotional states for internally modelling the mental states of other people. They are the consequence of reasoning logically from false premises about dispositions, motivations and intentions. This general process interacts with individual personality and circumstance to create specific delusional contents.

The conclusion would be that many of the social phenomena mentioned earlier (e.g. racism and strongly held political and religious views) can be conceptualised as operating with the same features of psychological organisation as delusional disorder. It is yet another example of the way in which emotions interact with cognition, so that perceptions are coloured by mood. Emotion shapes reasoning in a profound fashion, and because of the somatic marker mechanism, distinctive emotional colourings may be focused on particular social categories.

This is a way in which preconceptions may shape reasoning such that beliefs become almost unshakeable. When specific social categories become associated with certain classes of emotion, this constitutes what might be termed 'prejudice' in the exact sense of prejudging. If perceptions or recollections of Jewish or black people cause the enactment of aversive emotions, then these will affect the evaluations of social situations. A belief that 'the Jews' form a sinister, international conspiracy – powerful yet covert – may be strongly held, dominating, and in practice impossible to refute by argument. The belief is not illogical, but is based upon inference from indirect evidence.

Few people are immune to this kind of thinking, as the alternative to having strongly held beliefs on the basis of insufficient evidence is to have no strongly held beliefs at all, which is not an adaptive option – we *must* make judgements if we are to be socially competent. Something similar happens, I suggest, with other social categories, such as political parties. In a two-party political system there is a tendency to assume that one of the parties is basically well motivated although susceptible to mistakes, while the other party is basically wicked although capable of producing the occasional good policy, albeit for the wrong reason. People who support the same political party as I do are basically decent, while people who support the other party are basically selfish, stupid or misinformed. There is no neutral ground upon which this disagreement can be settled, and no way of determining which party really is the best, because all of the 'facts' are interpreted in the light of assumptions about motivations. It is no easier to persuade someone to change their political allegiance than it is to persuade someone with persecutory delusions that their beliefs are unfounded.

Although such social groupings as 'races', political parties or religions are so large and unorganised as to be abstract and amorphous, the structure of human intelligence is such that even when it is meaningless to attribute dispositions, intentions and motivations, human group categories gather to themselves emotions that are appropriately meant to be attached to individuals. As stated above, because we are social animals we must make judgements about who our allies are and who our enemies are – even when secure grounds for this decision are lacking and we cannot always tell the one from the other. However, for modern humans in mass societies the problem is impossible. We make judgements, and we stick by them and are dominated by them, even though that which we are judging is an artefact – a mere word that stands for something which may not exist, and which if it does exist may lack coherence and structure.

In effect, modern humans continue to anthropomorphise the social scene, and to personalise the impersonal, however inappropriate this may be. We naturally tend to turn everything into a 'human interest' story of heroes and villains, which is why tabloid journalists are so successful when they present issues in this way. However, having simplified life into a soap opera we become captives of our own assumptions and preconceptions. In this sense, delusional disorder is part of the human condition, and its importance increases with every passing year.

CHAPTER FIVE

Bizarre delusions

Two kinds of delusions – theory-of-mind delusions and bizarre delusions

Delusions, I suggest, fall into two categories, namely theory-of-mind delusions and bizarre delusions.

A theory-of-mind delusion is a false belief which is the logical outcome of a false premise. The processes of reasoning are intact and unimpaired, but are operating on incorrect assumptions. For Edward, the jealous murderer, two plus two still equals four and the sun still rises in the East. He remained able to give accurate accounts of direct observations of objective data. However, his assumption that his girlfriend was having an affair was based upon an incorrect interpretation of indirect inferences concerning her state of mind. Although her behaviour appeared to be consistent with the assumption of her sexual infidelity, the fact of the matter was that Edward's girlfriend was not actually having an affair.

However, false beliefs might also be the outcome of impaired thinking – of 'illogical' reasoning. Even correct premises would not necessarily lead to correct conclusions, as thinking is impaired. When reasoning is illogical, two plus two would not necessarily equal four, but might instead equal three, or five, or Adolf Hitler. The sun may rise in the West tomorrow, fail to rise at all, or have turned into a balloon.

Impaired thinking leads to bizarre beliefs

We are all familiar with this type of illogical reasoning that leads to bizarre delusions, as the illogical progression of ideas by association is the kind of thing that happens in dreams: 'I walked into the street and saw a lion and realised that to escape I needed to open a trapdoor hidden underneath the hedge, and the trapdoor opened on to another planet with purple skies and no gravity, but the lion had changed into a flowerpot. . .'

If we awaken from a doze, or are just dropping off to sleep, we may recall that our thoughts were 'falling apart' and becoming illogical. The release from a normal coherent progression to an unpredictable association of ideas varies in severity on a continuum from occasional mistakes to gross incoherence. The process can be observed from the outside when a delirious patient exhibits a fluctuating state of consciousness, with lucid intervals alternating with periods of incoherence.

Incoherent thinking and illogical reasoning are therefore often a consequence of 'clouded' consciousness or brain damage. And whenever thinking is impaired by 'organic' insult to the brain – for example, when consciousness is clouded, when we are sleepy, when the brain is reversibly impaired by drugs or alcohol or permanently impaired by dementia or other forms of brain damage – then under such circumstances there is a greatly increased potential for impaired reasoning to lead to false beliefs.

Beliefs resulting from illogical thinking can be extremely bizarre, especially since the mechanism for testing ideas for plausibility and consistency with other ideas is exactly what is damaged.

Bizarre beliefs – a sign of madness

All delusions are not the same. While false beliefs about other people (e.g. about sexual infidelity or persecution) can be seen as variants of normal behaviour and based on rational reasoning, other false beliefs are based on irrational thinking, and only occur in 'mad' people who are suffering from a general form of impairment of brain function, and who will exhibit a variety of symptoms. These are the bizarre delusions.

There has long been recognition, albeit vague, that some 'bizarre' beliefs have a different pathological significance to false beliefs that stem from misinterpretation of real phenomena. Bizarre beliefs are evidence of mental illness in a way that ToM delusions are not. Indeed, I suggest that it is a feature of bizarre beliefs of a delusional nature that they are *never* the only sign of mental illness, but that bizarre delusions are invariably part of a clinical picture which includes a range of other 'psychotic' symptoms, such as hallucinations, or illogical and incoherent speech (so-called 'thought disorder').

Bizarre delusions include many of the most typical delusions seen in classic 'schizophrenic' patients – for example, those 'primary' delusions in which a person suddenly becomes convinced of something false without any understandable logical link – 'the traffic-lights turned green and I knew I was the son of God' or 'my thoughts stopped and I realised that they were being drawn out of my head by X-rays'.

Some bizarre delusions arise from hallucinations or other abnormal bodily or mental experiences. For example, 'the voices' may have told the patient that he was the son of God, or he believes that the funny feelings in his belly were caused by a satellite. These are bizarre ways of explaining bizarre experiences, and both experience and explanation probably share a common source in brain impairment.

Bizarre delusions contrasted with theory-of-mind delusions

Subject matter of bizarre delusions – anything

While theory-of-mind delusions are always about social phenomena, bizarre delusions might be about anything – social or environmental, physical or metaphysical, natural or supernatural.

Bizarre beliefs may survive objective refutation

Theory-of-mind delusions stem from inferences concerning the mental states of other people – in other words, from indirect inferences about entities which are not directly observable. However, bizarre delusions may be held *despite* the evidence of direct observation.

Evidence that a normal person would find compelling is not necessarily persuasive to someone with bizarre delusions. Because the reasoning processes are impaired in bizarre delusions, a chain of argument that would usually be considered to represent conclusive evidence against a belief does not have the force it would usually have.

For instance, a person with psychotic depression and nihilistic delusions may believe that their internal organs have rotted away, leaving them hollow. Such a person is holding a belief in the existence of a state of affairs that is incompatible with human life, yet this 'fact' of the delusion being impossible is not regarded as compelling. Indeed, this kind of patient may deny that they are alive at all, which again contradicts what would be considered to be the possibilities of objective fact. After all, one does not hold conversations when one is dead.

Whatever the arguments or evidence that are brought to bear, the bizarre delusional belief may remain unshaken because when brain function is impaired we cannot follow logic, and so logical argument does not have the power to persuade.

Bizarre delusions are not encapsulated by social category

Theory-of-mind delusions are characterised by false beliefs confined to a particular social category – for example, when the deluded person is only jealous of his wife (but not his sister), or only afraid of the local drug Mafia (but not the Freemasons). However, since bizarre delusions are caused by impaired reasoning, such delusions are not confined to particular social categories, and delusional thinking is liable to be a feature of many domains of discourse.

Pure cases of bizarre delusions will not exist

While ToM delusions can occur as 'pure cases' in people who are otherwise normal, it would be predicted that there will be no pure cases of bizarre delusions. That is to say, there will be no cases of people who have an encapsulated bizarre delusion with otherwise wholly normal psychological functioning. In lay terms, all individuals with bizarre delusions will be overtly 'mad' or in some other way suffering from brain impairment leading to a variety of psychological symptoms bearing in mind that, as described in Chapter 6, the most sensitive method of detecting functional brain impairment is by serial electro-encephalogram (EEG) measurements.

To put it another way, bizarre delusions are assumed to be a consequence of impaired reasoning processes, and reasoning processes are assumed to be abnormal as a consequence of an organic brain impairment such as delirium or dementia. If delirium or dementia are present, then there will inevitably be a widespread impairment of brain function which will produce not just a single false belief, but a variety of psychological symptoms typical of that form of impairment. A delirious patient will not merely have a false belief, but will also exhibit impairment of concentration, altered mood, and poor performance on short-term memory tasks.

Thus it is firmly predicted that bizarre delusions would *only* be found as part of a psychiatric syndrome – never as pure cases.

Bizarre delusions are caused by organic brain impairment

The category of *bizarre* delusions is not explicable in terms of rationally misinterpreting normal perceptions on the basis of misattributed intentions, motivations or dispositions. Bizarre delusions either require that the patient is rationally misinterpreting pathological psychological features such as hallucinations, or else the actual thought processes are irrational due to pathology and the chain of inference is itself illogical (e.g. 'they threw an egg at my window, and this meant I was a homosexual, so I switched on my radio'). The chain of inference is illogical by normal standards of language as a medium of communication, although the story may well be explicable in terms of personally significant 'associations' in just the same way that dreams can make a kind of subjective sense.

The exact psychopathological mechanisms by which bizarre delusions arise cannot be known until the processes of normal, non-pathological thinking are understood. They are not understood at present – we just do not know the ways in which inferences are made. However, it is not debated that irrational thinking and abnormal psychological experiences are a common feature of *organic* brain disease such as delirium, epilepsy or dementia. In other words, if a brain is dysfunctional or damaged, then it is unsurprising that it cannot perform cognitive processing in the normal fashion. The same applies to sleep or near-sleep states. False beliefs are to be expected in circumstance where brain impairment has affected the cognitive processes by which beliefs are generated.

Although epilepsy and dementia may have a significant role to play in generating psychiatric illness, it is *delirium* that is the most interesting possible cause of bizarre delusions. This is because delirium is a concept of critical importance in the neo-Kraepelinian diagnostic system. Indeed, delirium could be described as the keystone of the whole nosology. If current concepts of delirium are inadequate, and if the keystone of neo-Kraepelinian nosology is defective, then the current classification of psychiatric disorders will collapse like a packhorse bridge crumbling into the chasm beneath it.

CHAPTER SIX

Delirium and brain impairment

Brain impairment is another fact of everyday life. Many people are brain impaired for much of the time – few will avoid impairment for very long – and a substantial number of people are impaired on a permanent basis. One of the critical concepts in psychiatry is that of reversible cognitive impairment – in other words, impairment of brain function without any permanent changes in structure. The most convenient term for clear-cut impairment of brain function is *delirium*. Other terms for delirium include acute organic syndrome and acute or toxic confusional state, or simply 'confusion'.

The causes of delirium are manyfold. As well as toxic levels of intoxication with alcohol or other 'drugs', delirium can be induced by withdrawal of alcohol and other intoxicating drugs (e.g. in delirium tremens). Children and elderly people may suffer delirium when running a high fever, after an operation or severe trauma, or after any significant 'insult' to the brain (e.g. an acute illness or trauma).

However, perhaps the most common type of delirium is the state between sleeping and waking in which 'hypnogogic' hallucinations can occur, and in which people may temporarily not know where they are or what day it is. A person dropping off to sleep may hear voices or noises, or see things, and the same thing may happen on waking (or being half-awake and suffering sensory deprivation in the dark). Who has not awoken to experience a bizarre (albeit transient) belief hanging over from a dream? These are 'normal' everyday experiences of psychotic phenomena, and they are due to reversible functional brain impairment.

The fact that delirium causes psychotic symptoms such as hallucinations and bizarre delusions has been well established for some centuries. But what is the definition of delirium? What is the threshold at which it can be diagnosed? The nature of this definition determines whether or not the psychotic symptoms in a particular patient can be attributed to dementia.

Definition of delirium

Traditionally, the term delirium has been reserved for only the most severe end of the spectrum, characterised by *disorientation* (i.e. not knowing what day it is, where you are, who you are or what is going on). The other feature of delirium is 'clouding' of consciousness, which is defined as drowsiness, reduced awareness of the environment, poor concentration and distractible attention – a state compatible with either sleepiness or excitable agitation.

This definition on the basis of disorientation is quite clear-cut, and prevents the over-diagnosis of delirium. However, this categorical 'yes or no' definition obscures the fact that brain impairment is a continuum, not simply something that is present or absent. Furthermore, to equate delirium with disorientation causes the problem of under-diagnosis of mild (but significant) delirium. More sensitive and objective measures, particularly those such as the electroencephalogram (which measures 'brainwave' electrical activity across the brain surface), demonstrate that delirium can occur in the absence of disorientation. Making the diagnosis of delirium depend upon disorientation produces false-negative results – in other words, apparently negative results for individuals who would have solid EEG evidence of delirium, but whose cognitive impairment is missed by the crude disorientation test.

The reality seems to be that delirium is not all of one kind, but that different impairments produce different symptoms and signs. Delirium tremens as a result of acute alcohol withdrawal often causes terrifying visual hallucinations (traditionally of pink elephants or snakes). However, psychedelic drugs may induce a delirium characterised by pleasant emotional and sensory experiences. Presumably these differences reflect the nature of the chemical insult, and also differences between the parts of the brain that they affect. However, both are still classifiable as delirium.

In summary, there is a need for a subclassification of delirium, as well as a redefinition, in order to diagnose the condition with greater sensitivity.

The critical role of delirium in neo-Kraepelinian diagnosis

If we recognise that delirium is common, varied in form, occurs along a continuum of severity, and is not restricted to people who are disorientated, then clearly the role of delirium in psychiatric illness needs to be re-evaluated. This is particularly important as it is known that delirium can lead to almost any kind of psychiatric abnormality. Because of the ability of the various types of delirium to generate multifarious psychotic symptoms, the early psychiatrists involved in classifying mental illness needed to differentiate between the presence and absence of delirium, because when it *was* present there was no mystery about the cause of psychotic symptoms (a globally malfunctioning brain will *obviously* produce abnormal cognitions of one kind or another).

However, if psychotic symptoms could occur in the absence of delirium, then this would represent a fascinating enigma – *a whole new category of diseases* – characterised by psychotic symptoms in clear consciousness. These were termed the 'functional psychoses' and consisted of schizophrenia, mania and depression (and, in the early days, 'paranoia' – a category that has been replaced by the delusional disorders). One could speculate that a great deal of the mystique surrounding the functional psychoses – the 'core syndromes' of psychiatry, the special preserve of psychiatrists, the heart of the discipline of psychopathology

– rests upon the single assertion that here we have syndromes characterised by psychotic symptoms in the absence of delirium. The whole edifice of modern psychology is balanced upon this assumption.

Yet the symptoms of delirium are strikingly similar to those of acute schizophrenia or mania. Emotions are perplexed, fearful, paranoid and labile; attention is distractible; speech may be jumbled and illogical; behaviour may be inappropriate; and hallucinations, persecutory delusions and other bizarre delusions may be common. Indeed, the presence of disorientation and 'clouding' of consciousness may be the *only* factors that differ between delirium and acute psychosis.

This is very important, namely that schizophrenia and delirium may be symptomatically identical, the only difference between them being the presence or absence of clouding of consciousness. However, even that criterion is not considered to make a decisive or clear-cut difference in all patients. Clouding can occur in what are diagnosed as acute psychotic states (mania or schizophrenia), and as suggested above the more subtle signs of mild delirium are very common in psychosis.

Thus it appears that in practice there may be no clinical difference at all between, say, mania and an agitated delirium, which is to say that mania and delirium are indistinguishable. Traditionally, organic psychoses (dementia, delirium, epilepsy, etc.) in which there is 'coarse' brain damage have been assumed to be qualitatively different from 'functional' psychoses such as schizophrenia and the affective disorders, in which brain damage is assumed to be much more subtle. The differential diagnosis is made on the basis not of clinical symptoms, but of the long-term prognosis. A delirious state is assumed to be short-lived and a consequence of physical illness or some other form of brain insult, whereas mania is assumed to be a mood disorder representing a disposition of the individual, and which may or may not lead to delirium as a secondary feature. This is probably quite true, but it serves to obscure the fact that an acute manic, schizophrenic or other psychosis often appears to be an episode of delirium. The reason for this delirium is a legitimate source of inquiry, but the fact that the state *is* delirium seems quite straightforward.

Thus if the presence of disorientation and clouding of consciousness are not sufficiently sensitive measures of delirium, then the boundaries between acute functional psychosis and acute organic states are breached. In other words, delirium is the key concept that stands at the boundary between 'organic' and 'functional' psychoses. This distinction forms the fundamental basis of the whole Kraepelinian and neo-Kraepelinian nosology. If the absence of delirium does *not* characterise the functional psychoses, then there is very little basis for the diagnostic categories, and the whole implicit aetiological distinction between mania and delirium is thrown into doubt.

But if acutely psychotic patients *are* delirious...

The whole of modern diagnostic practice therefore rests upon the definition of delirium. And if, as I have argued, the threshold for diagnosing delirium has been set at too insensitive a level, then the whole of modern diagnostic practice, and consequently a great deal of the research literature, requires substantial reappraisal. This is serious stuff.

For example, consider hallucinations, another of the classic symptoms of 'madness' when they occur in 'clear consciousness' – in other words, in the absence of delirium. Supposing, after all, consciousness is clouded and delirium is not absent. This would certainly solve a longstanding mystery concerning the mechanism by which hallucinations are produced. There is a considerable speculative literature which attempts to explain the psychological mechanisms by which auditory hallucinations occur. Ingenious though this literature is, I find it extremely unconvincing. Again, the main problem is that we do not have any convincing models of *normal* cognitive activity, so the task of explaining abnormal cognitive activity by reference to breakdowns in the normal process is an extremely long shot.

However, if patients with hallucinations are actually delirious, then there is no problem. Everyone knows that delirious patients hallucinate. Although we do not know exactly why they hallucinate, it is no great mystery. A damaged or deranged brain does things like this. We have experienced it ourselves when dropping off to sleep, or seen it in our children or grannies when they had a high fever.

This is perhaps very similar to how hypnagogic hallucinations would be if we were at a sustained level of consciousness that was poised at the verge of sleep – not quite falling asleep, and not quite becoming fully awake. Such an interpretation explains the distractibility, poor concentration and poor cognitive performance of actively hallucinating patients. It is not so much that such patients are 'attending to hallucinations' – as they are frequently described as doing – but rather that they are delirious. Like other delirious patients, they have a fluctuating and frequently impaired conscious level – indeed, this is taken to the extreme.

To summarise, a hallucinating person is partially dropping off to sleep, dreaming and then awakening, repeatedly, so that the dreams are remembered.

Testing the delirium theory of psychotic symptoms

If hallucinations in schizophrenia, mania and depression are actually caused by delirium, there is no need to posit any special or exotic mechanism for hallucinations. These are not 'functional psychoses' without organic features, but rather they are organic syndromes in which consciousness is at a level intermediate between 'clear' consciousness and the 'organic' level of impaired consciousness that has disorientation as its hallmark.

The proposition is readily testable, because it implies that any actively hallucinating patient will show brain changes compatible with delirium, and these changes should be detectable by electroencephalogram (EEG) or any other valid, sensitive and convenient measure of brain function. Similarly, in the case of bizarre delusions, and the phenomena of 'thought disorder' such as incoherent speech, thought-insertion or thought-stopping, these patients should exhibit delirium. A study of EEGs on actively psychotic patients is logistically difficult to perform. None the less, it may be worth the effort. Patients with hallucinations, bizarre delusions or thought disorder should exhibit EEG changes compatible with delirium. If they do not do so, then my theory is wrong.

EEGs exhibit a wide range of normal variations, so in order to detect EEG *changes* it would probably be necessary to perform serial measurements. Fluctuating conscious level is the key – the hallucinating patient dips into, and out of, dreams. The prediction is that if, for example, EEG measurements were taken both during the hallucinations, and following recovery from them (that is logistically difficult, but perfectly achievable given the time and resources), then there should be evidence of pathologically significant change during the psychotic episode. Since (as suggested below) it is probable that interference with working memory is the cause of symptoms, then EEG changes should be sought in the prefrontal cortex, especially the dorso-lateral (upper-outer) regions.

During the episode of hallucination there should be evidence of fluctuating conscious levels, and a correlation between the actual experience of hallucination and an immediately preceding dip in conscious level. By contrast, and as a possible control group, pure cases with theory-of-mind delusions would *not* be predicted to demonstrate EEG abnormalities, because they do *not* have abnormal brain function.

Clinical implications of the delirium theory of psychosis

EEG changes are currently the most sensitive markers of delirium, but EEGs are inconvenient, inaccessible and expensive, and some patients may be unable or unwilling to co-operate with the procedure. Thus it is important to generate data on the correlations between clinical symptoms and the objective measures of EEGs, so that the clinical symptoms may eventually be used as a guide to diagnosis and treatment.

The following suggestions are little more than hunches or intimations, but possible clinical criteria for delirium might include the known 'prodromal' affective changes which form part of the spectrum of impending delirium.

I suspect that a *fearful perplexity* may turn out to be the characteristic mood which is indicative of subtle functional impairment of the brain. Perplexity is the sense that something is amiss, but we do not know what. I suggest that perplexity might be indicative of a state in which there is something wrong with the brain, and the brain is able to sense this impairment, but due to its impairment (especially the fluctuating conscious level) the brain cannot work out what it is that is wrong. In other words, there is probably a defect in the operation of working memory, which is necessary for the conscious mental manipulation of representations involved in 'working out' the meaning of events. The prediction is that acutely psychotic patients will be perplexed as their general affect, although this may not apply to chronically psychotic patients when brain damage may also have damaged emotional expression.

Distractible attention is probably the first cognitive deficit to emerge with delirium. The patient cannot concentrate for very long on any single line of reasoning, and is readily diverted from any particular line of thought or attempted task. Poor attention also affects the laying down of memory. I suggest that attention deficits might emerge as the key basic psychological variable (or *sign*, since they are more apparent to an observer than to the patient). Neurologically, poor attention is probably also a consequence of disrupted working memory, with interruption to the progression of associated representations.

Perhaps the action of working memory is repeatedly being disrupted by micro-sleeps, producing lapses of attention and loss of the sustaining of cognitive representations upon which working memory depends. To speculate, sometimes the micro-sleeps could produce dreams (perhaps leading to hallucinations), sometimes they might lead to bizarre associations of ideas typical of 'dream logic' (perhaps leading to bizarre delusions), and sometimes they interrupt the train of thought (perhaps leading to thought-stopping or sudden changes of subject). Attention cannot be focused under these circumstances, but wanders according to the strength and novelty of the stimulus, leading to distractibility, and the associations of ideas which occur in states of clouded consciousness.

Implications for nosology

A picture is emerging which interprets the classic 'mad' symptoms of the 'functional psychoses' (schizophrenia, mania and psychotic depression) as being caused by delirium – clouding of consciousness. This stands in total contrast to the traditional view of 'functional psychoses' being *defined* as phenomena that occur in *clear* consciousness. The discrepancy is asserted to be due to an excessively insensitive definition of delirium and clouding.

However, even after this has been taken into account, it is important to note that although the functional psychoses are associated with delirium, it is delirium of a distinctive kind. After all, these are delirious people who have a remarkably high level of cognitive functioning. This leads us to ask about the pathological causes of delirium in those psychiatric diagnoses that are usually considered to be 'functional' rather than organic. The pathology must be reversible, because patients usually get better or at least improve substantially. The answer is presumably that acute psychotic states have the same types of pathology that can cause reversible delirium of other kinds. Exactly which kind has yet to be established, and would probably require specific enquiry in each patient.

In this context it is especially interesting to consider sleep deprivation. Chronic severe sleep deprivation is a feature of many psychotic patients, and whether this is a cause or an outcome of pathology (it could differ for different cases), chronic, severe sleep deprivation could certainly cause delirium. I shall be exploring the possible role of sleep deprivation in psychopathology in depression, mania and schizophrenia in the chapters devoted to those putative diagnoses.

In summary, then, hallucinations, bizarre delusions, thought disorder and other 'psychotic' phenomena are a consequence of delirium – and delirium is a state of reversibly impaired brain function which we have redefined in a more sensitive as well as scientifically objective fashion.

Delirium is therefore a basic phenomenon of psychiatry which occurs in many circumstances, and leads to many of the most striking psychiatric symptoms. The pathologies of psychotic delirium are simply the normal causes of cerebral impairment, and delirium is found with a wide range of severities, and interacting with individual differences in disposition to produce different clinical phenomena.

Psychiatric nosology will need to find a much larger place for delirium, a classification of the types of delirium, and scales for measuring its severity. A great deal of work needs to be done.

CHAPTER SEVEN

The 'anti-delirium' theory of electroconvulsive therapy (ECT) action

Having clarified the nature of delirium we can now approach some of the major phenomena of psychiatry with a fresh eye. It turns out that some of the longstanding enigmas of psychiatry are less enigmatic than is usually supposed. This applies not only to the diagnostic categories, but also to the major treatments. And of all the enigmas of psychiatry, the one that stands most in need of explanation and understanding is probably electroconvulsive therapy (ECT).

The mysterious nature of ECT

ECT is one of the most rapidly acting and powerful treatments used in psychiatry. Its effects on severe depression (melancholia) have been extensively documented, but ECT is also an effective therapy in many cases of mania, acute schizophrenia, delirium and Parkinson's disease. However, the lack of a convincing physiological rationale for its effectiveness has served to cast a cloud over the use of ECT in psychiatry, which is under endemic threat from those who perceive it to be intrinsically invasive and coercive.

ECT involves putting the patient to sleep with anaesthetic,

giving a muscle relaxant, applying electrodes to the scalp and inducing a *grand mal* epileptic fit by passing direct-current electricity through the brain at the minimum dose necessary to induce the seizure. The muscle relaxant prevents the patient from damaging him- or herself by violent movements during the fit. After the fit, the muscle relaxant quickly wears off, then the anaesthetic wears off and the patient awakens.

It is generally agreed that the therapeutic effect of ECT comes from the *grand mal* convulsion (rather than from the anaesthetic, the passage of electricity through the skull and brain, or other aspects of the manoeuvre). Thus any means of inducing a generalised epileptic seizure (e.g. by inhalation of camphor or injection of leptazol) is considered to be equally effective. ECT just happens to be the safest and most reliable means to this end.

This suggests that ECT action involves large volumes of brain tissue, since it is highly implausible that a generalised fit would have an extremely focused effect on a specific brain region. It also suggests that *the therapeutic action of ECT is 'simple'*, in the sense of working by its effect on basic biological variables such as arousal, rather than acting on specific regions or detailed aspects of brain function. Furthermore, any explanation of the effectiveness of ECT should account for the broad spectrum of diagnostic categories for which it is effective. As described above, the potential indications go beyond the most common usage of ECT in severe major depression with biological features.

I suggest that the primary therapeutic physiological effect of ECT is in the treatment of delirium, probably by simulating or inducing physiologically 'natural' and restorative sleep. The beneficial effect of ECT might be achieved either by the epileptic seizure itself mimicking sleep, or it might be caused by the 'post-ictal' sleep which occurs after an epileptic seizure. However, as clinical trials have demonstrated, the core therapeutic benefit of ECT certainly does not come from the use of anaesthesia. Anaesthesia is a state quite distinct from natural sleep.

One line of evidence in support of this view is that a course of ECT cumulatively leads to electroencephalogram

(EEG) changes characterised by increased amplitude and reduced frequency ('delta' activity). These changes produce an EEG trace somewhat similar to that seen in normal sleep. According to some research at least, it is likely that the presence of such EEG changes in a patient is correlated with improved clinical response to ECT and reduced likelihood of relapse.

The effects of ECT – a sleep surrogate or sleep-inducer

If the account of delirium as any significant functional brain impairment is accepted, it can be seen that by the time psychiatric patients are considered for ECT they will typically have suffered several months of altered sleep habit, amounting to chronic severe sleep deprivation (often combined with a shift in diurnal rhythm manifested in early-morning awakening). Significant impairment of brain function would be expected. It is possible that delirium secondary to sleep deprivation is the cause of the mental and physical slowing ('psychomotor retardation') that is a frequent and diagnostically important feature of major depression.

Severe sleep disturbance is also a feature of mania, in which a period of several days without any sleep at all often precedes an acute breakdown, and where inability or unwillingness to sleep is a major clinical symptom. In this respect, depression may resemble the somnolent form of delirium (characterised by EEG slowing) and mania may resemble the agitated form of delirium (characterised by rapid EEG traces). This prediction is readily susceptible to empirical testing.

In mania and delirium, even a single ECT treatment may serve to disperse an excited, insomniac, hyperactive state. When ECT is effective in depression, the patient often wakes from the first treatment feeling symptomatically improved, and further improvement may follow sound sleep during the following nights.

I suggest that ECT is a specifically effective treatment for depression *only* in those depressed patients who are at an advanced stage of their illness, and in whom delirium (and the putative delirium-related symptoms such as psycho-motor retardation, hallucinations and delusions) is a feature. Stressors such as insomnia and acute weight loss might also be expected to lead to changes in physiological and metabolic status which amount to a systemic illness with immune activation. As I have argued in the chapter on depression, the specific mood of depression may be a secondary consequence of a cytokine-mediated psycholo-gical and physical *malaise* including the typical pattern of 'sickness behaviour' (including demotivation, inertia, anhedonia, exhaustion, anorexia and sleep disturbance), and sleep deprivation might be expected to synergise with any pre-existing systemic illness in the production of delirium.

ECT breaks this vicious circle by inducing a generalised epileptic seizure which acts upon the brain like a deep and restorative sleep, the distinctive features of which require further investigation. It is possible that the *grand mal* is itself functionally akin to deep sleep, or it may be that the post-ictal state following the fit acts as a surrogate for sleep. Moreover, 'sleep' – in the sense of a physiologically restora-tive process – must be differentiated from 'unconsciousness'. It is clear from trials of 'sham' ECT that a general anaes-thetic alone is not equivalent to ECT in its specifically thera-peutic effect. This is also consistent with the lack of a subjectively restorative effect from general anaesthesia. Physiological sleep is clearly a more complex phenomenon than mere unconsciousness, and an ECT surrogate would need to replicate the physiological state of natural deep sleep.

Predictions

While ECT exerts its major effect on sleep, there may be other effects of the treatment. Indeed, it is usual for effective psychoactive interventions to have several actions, some useful and some unwanted. For example, it may be that repeated ECT may have effects, say, on entraining circadian rhythmicity (the sleep–wake cycle), or on raising the threshold to pain and other forms of aversive sensation, and these effects may result from quite different causes (e.g. hormone release). However, the effect on delirium seems to be the most striking and rapid action of ECT.

The sleep theory of ECT action makes several radical predictions. Most strikingly, and in contrast to current conceptualisations, ECT is *not* seen as a specifically antidepressant or mood-elevating intervention, despite being most commonly used as a treatment for severe depression. Indeed, as I shall argue in the chapter on depression, I do not regard any of the traditional antidepressants as being primarily active upon mood – mood is an end state or consequence of emotions, and not a primary psychological variable. The prediction is therefore that ECT should *not* be specifically effective (i.e. over and above placebo) when delirium is absent. This is consistent with ECT being more effective in late and severe depression in hospitalised populations than it is when used to treat early, mild or out-patient cases.

It seems probable that late depression has often entered a self-perpetuating, positive-feedback stage in which the original cause is no longer operating and the symptoms are mutually reinforcing and sustaining. Perhaps delirium maintains a pattern of insomnia and anorexia which, in turn, sustains delirium. The intervention of ECT breaks this positive feedback loop, clears delirium with deep sleep, resolves hallucinations and delusions, and allows a normalisation of sleep and appetite which restores physiological normality. Eventually mood recovers and stabilises.

Properly administered ECT with a confirmed *grand mal* seizure should be rapidly effective if it is going to be specifically effective. Cases which apparently only improve after many treatments over long periods of time would be expected to be responding to placebo effects, coincident therapeutic treatments (e.g. ongoing pharmacological or psychological therapies) or undergoing a natural remission. It would be predicted that if ECT responsivity was rigorously defined as only occurring in those patients with a rapid response (after one or two treatments), the presence of delirium (as defined by EEG) would be seen to be a major factor in defining the population that is likely to benefit from ECT.

Furthermore, improvement in 'delirious symptoms' such as psychomotor retardation, hallucinations and bizarre delusions may be immediate, but full resolution of the affective component of the illness would typically take longer. This staged improvement may be missed by the employment of generalised depression scales that measure global improvement in the depressive syndrome (such as those of Hamilton or Beck). Instead, clinicians should adopt a line of questioning directed at discovering the *first* signs of clinical improvement. (For instance, observers often notice objective improvements in activity, appetite or sleep several days before the patient reports an improvement in subjective mood.)

The delay in affective response to ECT may be explained by the general model according to which mood is a secondary consequence of cognitive functioning, and recovery of mood builds up following an accumulation of positive cognitions. Sleep patterns and appetite are restored, and gradually the accumulated exhaustion of several months is repaired. Just as full recovery from influenza takes a few weeks, so the process of recovery from depression (which probably shares many common phenomenological and possibly pathological features with influenza) would be expected to proceed over a similar time scale.

It seems that ECT is not primarily or specifically an antidepressant treatment. Instead, it exerts its therapeutic effects on mood indirectly by simulating or inducing deep sleep to resolve delirium. Subjectively satisfying and objectively physiologically normal sleep is not always easily attained by pharmacological means, and 'hangover' effects from sedatives may cause troublesome daytime somnolence which further disrupts circadian rhythms, yet the benefits of sleep may be rapid and profound. If a less invasive substitute for ECT were desired, the priority would be to devise an equally powerful and rapid means of inducing physiologically restorative sleep.

CHAPTER EIGHT

The malaise theory of depression

Depression – the need for a fundamental reappraisal

Depression is probably the commonest of the formally diagnosed psychiatric illnesses – 'the common cold of psychiatry'. Certainly depression is so frequent as to be a substantial element in the human condition. Many people will be diagnosable as depressed at some point in their lives, and almost everyone will have a close relative or friend who suffers from depression. And the diagnosis and treatment of depression is one of the great success stories of post-war psychiatry – with greatly improved detection of the disorder and a wide range of effective antidepressant interventions available that have enormously improved the outcome.

None the less, depression is not well understood. The word 'depression' itself presents a problem. There is continued confusion in the mind of the general public about the relationship of 'everyday' sadness to the syndrome of 'major depressive disorder' (MDD). Within MDD is a huge range of severity, from patients who are able to hold down a job and function at a high level to those who do not eat or drink, cannot speak or move and are candidates for emergency ECT. The syndromal diagnosis of MDD does not explain what depression *is* – it merely offers a thumbnail sketch of the kind of person who gets diagnosed as suffering from MDD – and these individuals show extraordinarily wide variation.

To exacerbate matters further, there is a problem in explaining how antidepressant drugs work – that is, in explaining why a chemical is apparently sometimes the best way of removing sadness and restoring a 'normal' mood state. No amount of proof of the effectiveness of antidepressants or ECT seems to be able to remove the suspicion that surrounds these treatments (especially among the more highly educated part of the population, who persistently favour psychological explanations and treatments of depression, even when these are wholly lacking any specific evidence base). The usual 'scientific' explanations of antidepressant action suggest that levels of specific brain chemicals are abnormal in depression (e.g. low levels of brain serotonin), and argue that this situation is corrected by antidepressants (a few of which supposedly have a specific influence on brain serotonin levels). Such theories are probably untrue, and certainly unproven.

The 'abnormal brain chemistry' story is also more frightening to lay people than most psychiatrists realise. Brain damage is one of the most dreaded conditions. To say that someone has an abnormal brain chemistry is to say they have brain damage – albeit mild and temporary – and this is probably even more stigmatising and scary than the lay explanation that depression occurs as a consequence of stresses and vulnerabilities. Ask yourself whether *you* would employ, or leave your children with, or marry, someone who has 'abnormal brain chemistry'. It sounds terrifying – how could such people be responsible for their actions? So, though the neurotransmitter story removes blame from patients, it also removes rationality. And if depression is reclassified from a response to misfortune to a form of reversible brain damage, then antidepressants are seen as mind manipulators – an equally scary notion.

Of course, in reality, many depressed patients are able to perform daily work and parenting to a high level, and to sustain human relationships; and the demonstrated effects of antidepressants on brain neurotransmitters are weak or perhaps even non-existent.

None the less, it is hardly surprising that, despite a mass of would-be common-sense and demystifying propaganda, the public remains frightened and unconvinced by the prevailing explanation of depression – what it is, what is wrong, and how antidepressants work. It is time for a fundamental reappraisal of the nature of depression.

The nature of mood and emotions

Major depression is one of the 'affective' or 'mood' disorders, which are psychological illnesses that are considered to have mood changes as their core symptom. Yet despite this central role of mood in psychiatry, mood itself is poorly conceptualised. What is mood? Is it a cause or an effect of behaviour? How is it represented in the brain? How does it interact with other forms of cognition? And what kind of a thing *is* mood? Before attempting to unravel the nature of depression and major depressive disorder, it is important to establish some conceptual clarity about affect.

As a starting point, mood has something to do with emotions. However, according to my understanding of contemporary cognitive psychology, mood is *not* a primary variable of psychological life. Sadness is not like fear. Rather, sadness is an end-product – not a primary cause but a secondary *consequence* of other variables, particularly of emotions. Although moods are recognised by characteristic facial expressions, brain centres for emotions such as fear and disgust have been found, but not brain centres for happiness or sadness. Fear and disgust are emotions; happiness and sadness are moods.

I suggest that mood is and should be used as nothing more than a summary term. To say a depressed person 'is sad' has no more depth or significance than to say that summer 'is warmer' than winter. Terms such as happiness, sadness and perplexity implicitly represent an average of a subjective state over a period of time. A person's 'mood' might be conceptualised as shorthand for the modal or mean average of their emotional states with respect to the very general categories of gratification or aversion, pleasure or pain, attraction or repulsion, action or inaction, or exploration or withdrawal.

There are two possible ways to have a 'depressed' mood – to be sad all the time, or never to be happy. Thus a person with a depressed mood might be someone whose usual mood is misery, or alternatively someone whose range of emotions is shifted such that they very seldom feel gratified. Similarly, a winter day is usually colder than a summer day, and even on the hottest winter day it never gets as warm as the hottest summer day. Happiness is therefore just a word used to summarise the many ways in which a person may experience gratification as their usual emotion, while sadness is a term used for the state caused by aversive emotions. The ascription of mood does no more than indicate the characteristic emotion.

A person's characteristic emotion will define a characteristic 'cognitive style', a way of interpreting and responding to stimuli. The happy man sees a different world to the world of the unhappy man. Each of them attends to different stimuli, their perceptions are processed differently, and they show different responses to the same stimuli.

Depression is not a valid aetiological category, nor does it describe a unified cause. Rather, the term 'depression' describes an end-state, a characteristic emotional *range*. More precisely, depression is a state of the body (and mind) that is composed of other more primary emotions. There are as many causes of 'depression' (in the sense of sadness or misery) as there are causes of aversive states, and there are as many ways of being sad and miserable as there are differences in personality and experience. Therefore there is no clear single category relating to the *mood* of depression, sadness or misery. One person's low mood may be entirely different in cause and quality to any other. One person may be fearful and anxious, another may feel hopeless, a third may be subject to severe downward mood swings, and a fourth may be 'unable to feel'. All of these and other types of misery may represent different pathologies, rather than being 'subtypes' of depression.

However, among this potentially limitless diversity of negative human states, there does appear to be a specific syndrome which is approximated by the diagnostic category of major depressive disorder. I suggest that MDD is a cross-culturally observed syndrome which forms a reasonable basis from which to look for an illness with a genuine psychological unity. I shall argue that MDD is not an affective category (i.e. it is not a 'mood disorder'), but instead it is a behavioural syndrome that approximates to a legitimate unified and underlying biological 'core' emotional state that will be termed *malaise*.

Deficiencies in current understanding

My stance will be that the diagnostic syndrome of MDD is broadly along the right lines. However, MDD should not be considered as an 'affective disorder' (an illness *primarily* of mood). Instead, MMD should be reinterpreted as summarising the behavioural outcome of a unified aversive malaise state called 'sickness behaviour' that is caused mainly by immune chemicals such as cytokines.

One problem with conceptualising MDD as an affective disorder is that there is no consistent affect. Many MDD patients deny that they feel sad or miserable, and the diagnostic schemas (such as DSM-IV and ICD-10) specify a variety of supposedly 'characteristic' mood states such as hopelessness, 'anhedonia' (reduced or absent capacity to experience pleasure), anxiety, distress and irritability. This variety of dissimilar moods seems excessively imprecise for a primarily 'affective' diagnostic category.

It has proved difficult to conceptualise how 'sadness' could constitute an illness, and even harder to understand how ingesting a simple chemical could specifically alleviate sadness and restore normal 'euthymic' mood. Antidepressants are not euphoriants like amphetamine, nor do they intoxicate like MDMA ('ecstasy'), nor are they considered to be addictive or dependence-inducing (recreational abuse is very rare). So what antidepressants do *not* do is well established, yet their positive psychological action remains obscure. In addition, antidepressants are commonly supposed to have a delay of two to six weeks before the onset of therapeutic action. If this is true, it would make antidepressants unique in the whole of pharmacology, as even the slowest of other agents (e.g. hormones that affect DNA transcription, such as cortisol or thyroxine) have a measurable onset of action within just a few days.

The problem here is that, since the psychological nature of depression is unclear, the way in which antidepressants act upon depression is also unclear.

Emotions and the somatic marker mechanism

When emotions reflect pathological states, they can have damaging effects on behaviour – in this case, emotions are maladaptive. For example, fear is adaptive when fight or flight is appropriate. However, if a person's physiological state of fear is excessive, or without adequate cause – when fear is pervasive and chronic rather than being related to specific dangerous situations – then the emotion is no longer a good guide to behaviour. In such pathological states, a person may be described as being *locked into* the emotion. When an individual is locked into a pathological emotional state the emotion is not activated when needed and as appropriate, but instead distorts behaviour in ways that may be unpleasant and/or harmful.

When it is pathological, fear becomes associated with all perceptions instead of just those that are potentially dangerous. We do not just experience fear on seeing a lion, but also on perceiving a mouse. This inappropriate fear feeds into working memory and interacts with perceptions by the somatic marker mechanism. These perceptual–emotional representations are stored in long-term memory.

The here-and-now primary emotions of which we are aware are fearful, and this means that incoming perceptions are interpreted as anxiety-provoking (i.e. we feel fear and 'therefore' infer that the stimuli in our environment must be frightening us). However, the effect of being locked into a state of fear also influences secondary emotions via the somatic marker mechanism. When we recall perceptual information from long-term memory, the cognitive representation also causes us to re-experience the emotional state that was laid down with it. Thus when fear-marked cognitions are laid down as long-term memories, they accumulate to become a *disposition* or characteristic way of appraising and reacting to the world. More and more things become fear-provoking to us.

If a person in a state of anxiety sees a mouse, then the somatic marker mechanism may record the anxiety along with the memory of the mouse. When the identity of the mouse is recalled from long-term memory, then these memories may be perceived as fear-provoking. We think of a mouse, and the fear which 'marked' this representation is re-enacted in our body.

Thus memories that are laid down when a person is locked into a pathological emotional state may become coloured by that emotion. If the emotion was fear, then anticipated situations evoke dread. In this way long-term psychiatric illness cumulatively affects personality by impressing characteristic emotional states on to the content of long-term memory.

However, whatever the original *causes* of fear in the past or present, anxiolytic drugs may be effective in alleviating the *physical* state of current anxiety, diminishing the manifestations of fear. For example, propranolol may act to diminish the peripheral manifestations of anxiety such as accelerated heart rate, and diazepam may diminish muscular tension. This reduces the primary emotion of fear in the here and now, as it is interpreted by the brain on the basis of monitoring the state of the body. However, the secondary emotion of fear is also affected. So we think of the mouse, and recall to awareness in working memory the long-term memory that contains both perception and emotion, but we do not feel anxious because the anxiolytic drug blocks the bodily response to this memory. The anxiolytic agent prevents the body from enacting the emotion of fear – therefore the heart rate does not increase, we do not break into a sweat, and our muscles do not become tense.

In other words, anxiolytics treat the *proximate* mechanisms of fear – that is, the mechanisms by which fear is physically manifested. I shall argue that the situation with regard to fear and anxiolytics finds a close parallel in the situation relating to major depressive disorder and antidepressants. Antidepressants block the proximate mechanisms that cause the characteristic emotion of depression.

Major depressive disorder is sickness behaviour

The emotional state of 'depression' can be approached in a manner closely analogous to the emotional state of fear, which is so well characterised – in other words, by seeking the adaptive function of the pattern of behaviour termed 'major depressive disorder', elucidating the factors which mediate these behaviours, and analysing the ways in which pharmacological and other interventions might have beneficial effects on different components of the system. Anxiety in humans can be seen as equivalent to fear in other animals since they share an identical biochemical, physiological and behavioural pattern. Similarly, MDD in humans has its biochemical, physiological and behavioural equivalent in other species.

Remarkably, it turns out that the syndrome of MDD is virtually identical with a syndrome seen in animals. The animal equivalent of MDD is the adaptive state termed *sickness behaviour* (SB). Sickness behaviour is the characteristic behaviour pattern of a sick animal, and was first described by a veterinarian as a physiological and psychological adaptation to acute infective and inflammatory illness in many mammalian species. Major depressive disorder is sickness behaviour that is inappropriately activated or excessively sustained.

The characteristic pattern of sickness behaviour consists of pyrexia, fatigue, somnolence, psychomotor retardation, impaired cognitive functioning and demotivation with regard to normal drives such as appetite for food and sex (this probably corresponds to anhedonia in humans, which is the inability to experience pleasure). In other words, the syndrome of SB is almost exactly the same as the standard diagnostic descriptions of MDD. The only apparent differences, namely somnolence and pyrexia, are explicable given that daytime somnolence typically leads to secondary insomnia and nocturnal sleep disruption, and that the presence of pyrexia has not been evaluated in MDD (it may be that patients with MDD do have a raised temperature in the early stages of the illness, but that this state has resolved by the time they are seen by psychiatrists or are admitted to hospital).

The evolved function of SB is to act as an energy-conserving, risk-minimising, immune-enhancing state appropriate for a body mounting a short-term, all-out attack on an invading micro-organism. MDD is therefore the behavioural response to a physical illness – it is a syndrome in which low mood is the product of *malaise*, where malaise describes the symptom of 'feeling ill'. By this account, the feeling of malaise should be regarded as the *core emotion* of depression.

Malaise is an emotion because it is based upon a characteristic physiological disposition as represented in the brain. In other words, the brain receives feedback about certain aspects of the body state, especially the presence of increased concentrations of circulating cytokines and similar immune products, and interprets these as evidence of sickness requiring adaptive behavioural changes to conserve energy, minimise risk and fight the disease.

Therefore MDD is not primarily an affective disorder – the syndrome is not driven by a change in mood. Instead, the primary pathology in MDD is somatic (i.e. of the *body*), and mood is a secondary and variable response to this disordered physical state. The major psychological change involves an emotion (i.e. malaise) rather than a mood (e.g. sadness).

Cytokines as mediating factors in sickness behaviour

The emotion of fear is mediated by the sympathetic nervous system. The analogous mediating factor for depression appears to be hyperactivity of the immune system in response to 'non-self' antigenic challenge (e.g. inflammation due to infection, carcinoma or 'autoimmune' disease). The chemical factors responsible for mediating sickness behaviour appear to be the class of immune-active agents known as *cytokines* (e.g. interleukins and interferons). Indeed, SB is best regarded as an integral and adaptive part of the pyrexial response. SB is the behavioural change that aids in the generation and maintenance of raised body temperature, and is appropriate to general immune activation.

There is abundant evidence to support the contention that malaise is mediated by cytokines. For instance, administration of cytokines to mammals provides a model for depression. An intravenous infusion of interferon into humans rapidly produces a syndrome that is psychologically and physically identical to MDD. Moreover, the high incidence of depression and other aversive psychiatric side-effects is well recognised as perhaps the most significant clinical limitation on the therapeutic use of cytokines such as interferon for the treatment of cancer and viral infections.

One important aspect of cytokines is that they produce *hyperalgesia* or increased sensitivity to pain. This provides a plausible mechanism for generation of the physical symptoms of depression, and possibly contributes to the related illness of chronic fatigue syndrome. Ordinary bodily sensations, which would usually be ignored, rise above the threshold of awareness when cytokines are circulating. These aversive sensations, which really have no pathological significance, are then perceived as pains, aches, heaviness and fatigue. Like all aversive signals, they are difficult to ignore because the body interprets them as a warning of pathology, usually altering the motivational state in the direction of rest and immobilisation.

The clinical evidence for cytokines being the cause of MDD is also compelling, as there is a substantial literature documenting significant immune activation in depression, with a wide range of abnormalities in cytokines and other acute-phase proteins, correlating with the natural history of the illness and response to therapy. It would be predicted that cytokine abnormalities would be even clearer and more specific if studies were restricted to only those 'depressed' patients who exhibited the syndrome of sickness behaviour with prominent symptoms of malaise.

As something of a sideline, there may also be an interesting relationship between cytokines and the 'stress-hormone' system. The major stress hormone is cortisol, which is secreted by the adrenal gland. Some of the cytokines have a direct action in stimulating the secretion of adrenocorticotrophic hormone (ACTH), which in turn stimulates cortisol. The latter is a powerful anti-immune and anti-inflammatory agent (cortisol or its analogues are often used for this purpose as a drug). What appears to be happening is that cortisol provides a negative feedback effect on cytokines, in suppressing their secretion and their immune effects.

Many depressed patients have raised blood levels of cortisol, and it is plausible that the raised cortisol concentration is actually doing these patients some good, at least in the sense of diminishing some of the symptoms of raised cytokine levels. For example, cortisol has actions as a painkiller or analgesic, and this would be expected to combat (to some extent) the hyperalgesic effects of cytokines. Terminally ill patients with widespread malignancy are often given steroids to improve their mood and sense of well-being. Furthermore, many patients with symptoms of chronic fatigue appear to have raised blood cytokine levels but *without* raised blood cortisol. Raised cytokine levels but no cortisol analgesia might explain why chronic fatigue patients may suffer extreme symptoms of fatigue – they are suffering from the 'unopposed' action of cytokines. This suggestion is consistent with reports that chronic fatigue responds to low (i.e. physiological rather than pharmacological) doses of cortisol analogues.

The bizarre conclusion seems to be that patients with chronic fatigue syndrome characterised by raised cytokine levels may be a subtype of 'cortisol-deficient' MDD – and the addition of small doses of cortisol may make them simply depressed (but without the overwhelming fatigue). This predication is so odd that it just might be true. Time will tell.

Having suggested the primary somatic (physical) pathology of MDD, the 'characteristic' psychological changes of this syndrome now need to be explained. What causes the depressed mood?

Mood changes are secondary to sickness behaviour

Although animals demonstrate sickness behaviour mediated by cytokines in the same way as humans, only conscious animals such as humans can suffer from the distinctive 'existential' state of depression, with feelings such as nihilism, worthlessness, guilt and suicidal ruminations. The locked-in state of malaise which prevails in sickness behaviour interacts with memories of the past and anticipations of the future such that a demotivated, exhausted and profoundly dysphoric state of malaise fills and colours the past, present and the anticipations of future mental life.

Imagine a depressed person sitting on the edge of their bed, trying to get going. They think of breakfast, but have no appetite. Should they go for a walk? They feel exhausted. They are troubled by aches, pains and heaviness that force themselves on awareness. Might this be evidence of disease, maybe cancer? How about visiting a friend? On recollecting the last conversation there is no sense of pleasure – what might they talk about today? There is guilt because they should be eating, they should be exercising, they should go and see their friend, but... Whatever can be imagined fails to produce a stirring of pleasant anticipation, and the dull state of malaise continues.

Something like this is the state of a person with MDD, and describing it precisely in terms of mood is difficult (especially when one is demotivated and cannot see the point of making the effort). It may be described as sad and miserable in one sense, but also dull, unresponsive and 'nothing', because nothing seems to make a difference – action is tiring and unrewarding, and inaction merely allows more time for brooding and feeling the unpleasant state of one's own body.

Prolonged sickness behaviour therefore creates a nihilistic mental state in which life seems devoid of gratifying possibilities (i.e. pessimism prevails) because feedback registers a physiological state that is locked into SB and unresponsive to the usual appetites (i.e. anhedonia). Sufferers cannot 'pull themselves together' or 'snap out of it' any more than people with influenza can think themselves back to normal, or be cured by psychotherapy. Talking to a sick person may help to make them feel better, and it may improve their overall condition, but they will still be sick.

Another point is that, unlike the flu sufferer, the SB sufferer *does not know that they are sick*, and often interprets their lack of energy, lack of motivation and poor concentration as a *moral* failure, leading to feelings of guilt and unworthiness. And, of course, although it is overwhelmingly real ('no, I do not feel well, I feel sick'), the physical state is vague, hard to formulate, difficult to localise and pin down. This may even be exacerbated by the fact that psychiatrists are not interested in the sufferer's physical symptoms, never ask about them, and always explain them away as being secondary to mood. Given the nature of this subjective mental landscape, the high rate of suicide among individuals with MDD is unsurprising.

To put malaise at the core of the depressive syndrome may seem a radical inversion of the usually accepted causal interpretation, as symptoms of malaise have traditionally been interpreted as secondary to the mood change in MDD. Traditionally (e.g. in DSM-IV) it is supposed that depressed people complain of tiredness and aching limbs because they are miserable, whereas the malaise theory suggests that they are miserable because they are tired and have aching limbs, until eventually chronic misery is learned and becomes habitual, so that it may persist even after resolution of the SB.

However, to emphasise the physical symptomatology of the depressive is more of a re-emphasis than a novel discovery. Kurt Schneider (1959) considered the physical or 'vital' symptoms of depression to be of paramount diagnostic importance, and the nearest approach to a 'first-rank symptom' of affective disorders. Most comprehensive textbooks of psychiatry or psychopathology describe a range of typical 'depressive' physical symptoms such as exhaustion, washed-out feelings, aching, heaviness or pain. The malaise theory of depression suggests that Schneider's tentative hints were correct, and that a more coherent and biologically valid concept of depression can be created with these physical symptoms as the unifying primary psychopathology, and affective changes as a secondary, contingent and variable consequence.

Implications of the malaise theory of depression

If sickness behaviour is equivalent to major depressive disorder, this implies that instead of 'sad' mood being regarded as the primary symptom of MDD, the state of *malaise* should be seen as the core symptom of MDD.

Depressed people are *physically sick but do not know it*. Because they do not know it, depressed people blame themselves for their symptoms. 'Why am I so exhausted and doing nothing? Because I am useless, have no moral fibre, I am a failure as a husband, a bad father.'

This interpretation immediately suggests that knowledge of causes might have some therapeutic benefits for the depressed patient. To know that one is physically ill as a cause of malaise does not cure the problem, any more than knowing that one had influenza removes the physical suffering. However, even if such knowledge does not make you feel less *ill*, it may make the state of malaise less depressing.

As suggested above, past research into depression would need to be reinterpreted in the context of this new and *more restrictive* definition of major depressive disorder. According to the concept of MDD as SB, most previous studies of 'depression' can be seen to have contained heterogeneous diagnostic groups consisting of a mixture of some subjects with malaise and the other typical features of SB, and other subjects with few or no such features.

Because the malaise theory of depression has so many implications, it is readily testable. One startling implication is that the brain need not have any pathological involvement in the core syndrome of MDD (this may explain why robust evidence of a specifically depression-related cerebral pathology has proved elusive). It requires a profound conceptual shift to recognise that the syndrome of MDD may be the response of a 'healthy brain' to a 'sick body', especially in view of the hundreds of millions of pounds spent on the search for a pathognomonic brain lesion in depression. Although, of course, the brain may also be involved in any generalised inflammatory, immune or neoplastic pathology which is also associated with sickness behaviour, and any change in motivational behaviour must be associated with changes in the brain; in the minimal or 'core' state of MDD the brain merely monitors, interprets and responds behaviourally to a pathological change in the body.

The cognitive impairment seen in 'non-psychotic' MDD (i.e. characterised by symptoms such as poor concentration, reduced performance on short-term memory tasks, etc.) is not qualitatively distinct from the psychological symptoms which commonly occur in acute physical illnesses such as colds and flu, and colds and flu are not usually described as being associated with neurotransmitter abnormalities.

However, in the most severe and sustained cases of 'psychotic' MDD the brain is involved as well as the body. In such cases of brain involvement, qualitative cognitive impairment is found (e.g. psychomotor retardation, poor concentration and memory, hallucinations and delusions). These symptoms can be interpreted as instances of *delirium* (i.e. functional, reversible brain impairment). This cerebral pathology might occur either as a secondary consequence of generalised immune activation from a generalised pathology, or as a consequence of SB-specific factors such as chronic, severe sleep deprivation and perhaps starvation and dehydration. It would be predicted that MDD patients with psychotic symptoms would show abnormalities on EEG, especially slowing relative to the EEG in the non-psychotic state. Psychotic MDD patients are most effectively treated by electroconvulsive therapy (ECT), and this is understandable on the basis that ECT may function as a sleep-surrogate and antidelirium intervention, rather than acting primarily as an 'antidepressant'.

Autoimmune disease suggested as a cause of depression

The malaise theory leads to a variety of immunological predictions. One helpful aspect is that this theory points towards a useful animal model of depression, namely animals treated with cytokines to produce sickness behaviour. This could be very useful, as the lack of animal models of psychiatric disease has been a very important barrier to the development of new drugs.

There is also a need for more precise understanding of the complex cytokine changes associated with sickness behaviour in humans. In particular, we need to search for any causal relationships between specific patterns of immune abnormality and specific psychological symptoms. For instance, specific cytokine abnormalities may cause specific psychological symptoms.

Alternatively, psychological causes could trigger physical change. In *The Suspended Revolution* David Healy (1990) pointed out the clinical similarity between 'jet lag' and major depressive disorder. It is probable that any cause of significant sleep deprivation or disruption in sleep-wake cycles would be a cause of endocrine stress and therefore potential immune system changes. Sleep disruption is a plausible final common pathway for many potentially depression-precipitating 'life events' such as bereavement.

There is also the possibility of monitoring the depressive illness biochemically. Longitudinal changes in cytokines (or their surrogate indices, e.g. C-reactive protein) would be expected to mirror the progress and activity of MDD. Hence cytokine monitoring may provide a marker of treatment response, or serve as a marker of remissions and relapses. Some depressed patients may actually be pyrexial, or exhibit more subtle abnormalities of the diurnal rhythm of body temperature, especially in the early stages of the illness.

However, perhaps the most important contribution that immunologists could make would be to elucidate the nature of the 'hyper-immune states' that are associated with MDD. What are the primary causes of MDD? It is likely that there are as many causes of MDD as there are causes of sickness behaviour, but it may also be that 'classic' MDD as seen by psychiatrists will correspond to a more specific pathological state.

The natural history of classic, psychiatrist-observed MDD is of a reversible illness with a natural history of several months, eventually leading to a spontaneous remission and typically full recovery. Some people are more prone to this illness than others. Patients with a family history of MDD, or a past history of MDD, have an increased probability of relapse. This pattern of natural history and epidemiology is reminiscent of some of the 'autoimmune' diseases akin to rheumatoid arthritis.

It would therefore seem worthwhile to test the idea that 'classic' cases of MDD may be caused by some kind of 'autoimmune' disease, namely a relapsing and remitting inflammatory disease which produces increased secretion of cytokines. Certainly the typical natural history is similar to that seen in a number of the autoimmune diseases (e.g. rheumatoid arthritis), with a typical time scale of weeks or months per episode, spontaneous recovery between episodes, and so on.

An autoimmune cause of MDD might explain the inherited genetic predisposition and the MDD trait such that one episode predicts an increased likelihood of others. Individual inflammatory episodes might then be triggered by a variety of environmental, pathological, behavioural or developmental factors, as with rheumatoid arthritis. All of this is highly speculative, but some cases of MDD might end up being classified with the 'connective-tissue diseases'.

Conclusion

It is important to emphasise that although sickness behaviour is an evolved, adaptive response to infection, MDD is a *maladaptive* manifestation of sickness behaviour. The analogy is with generalised anxiety – although fear is an adaptive behavioural pattern, when fear is *continuously activated* it becomes pathological.

Similarly, when sickness behaviour occurs as a short-term response to acute infection it is (on average) adaptive and may be life-saving. However, when SB is activated continuously and outside the circumstances for which it evolved, it is of course dysfunctional. In an acute infectious illness, the state of demotivation is valuable in that it conserves energy for an all-out fight against infection. However, when sickness behaviour is sustained or inappropriately evoked, this long-term state of demotivation will be profoundly damaging – after all, animals must eventually eat and reproduce.

Thus MDD, although it is an evolved behavioural pattern, is indeed maladaptive and dysfunctional – in a nutshell, it is pathological. MDD should continue to be considered an illness, and undoubtedly one of the worst. Knowing that MDD is primarily a physical illness may of itself be therapeutically beneficial. However, the main role of the malaise theory is to improve treatment – and that is the next topic for consideration.

Antidepressant drug action

If major depressive disorder is sickness behaviour, and depressed mood is best conceptualised as malaise due to physical illness, then what is the action of antidepressants and how do they improve depressed mood? In the first place, we must distinguish between specifically antidepressant drugs which act on malaise, and drugs that might be helpful in some other way in a depressive illness.

I suggest that, since malaise is seen as the core symptom of depression, then a *specifically* antidepressant drug should have as its primary action the alleviation of malaise and the other 'vital' physical symptoms of MDD, such as fatigue, heaviness, aches and pains. Of course, psychiatric drugs are relatively non-specific, as are current diagnoses, and drugs other than specific antidepressants may be valuable in the treatment of other aspects of the MDD syndrome. For example, benzodiazepines may alleviate symptoms such as insomnia or anxiety, and neuroleptic drugs may help with hallucinations and delusions experienced in association with depression. However, the *core* activity of antidepressants should relate to the core symptoms of depression – that is, the primary, syndrome-creating physical symptoms associated with malaise.

When cytokine-induced fatigue, demotivation, aches and pains occur during acute infectious diseases such as influenza, these symptoms are usually treated by *analgesia*. For example, people usually take aspirin or paracetamol when they have flu – partly to bring their temperature down, and partly to relieve aching and washed-out feelings. I suggest that, in this sense, *true antidepressants are analgesics*, on the basis that any drug which alleviates subjectively dysphoric states can be considered to be an analgesic.

My assertion is that antidepressants are drugs whose specifically antidepressant action is the treatment of an aversive physical state to make patients feel better – very much as aspirin can make patients with flu feel better. In other words, antidepressants are *anti-malaise analgesics*. When patients feel less 'sick', their mood will (usually) start to improve, just as people usually start to feel more cheerful after they have recovered from flu. Thus antidepressants do not 'make people happy', but (when effective) they remove a significant obstacle to happiness. It is easier to be happy in the absence of malaise, although happiness is certainly not guaranteed.

Conceived in this fashion, the anti-malaise analgesic effect of antidepressants on mood is no more remarkable than the fact that it is easier to be happy without a chronic headache than with one. This is the simple answer to the puzzling fact that a chemical such as an antidepressant can apparently treat so complex a thing as human misery. The true antidepressant is not a mind-manipulating drug, nor is it a 'happy pill'. Antidepressants could be regarded as a kind of 'mood aspirin'. When it is effective, an antidepressant can alleviate aversive symptoms of pain and sickness, and give people a better chance of enjoying life.

Antidepressants as analgesics

There is conclusive evidence to support the idea that tricyclic antidepressants act as analgesics when tested in both human and animal models. Tricyclics are increasingly used in the management of chronic pain, neurogenic pain, migraine, chronic fatigue, cancer pain, AIDS and arthritis. I suggest that analgesia is not just a fortunate side-effect of tricyclics, but that it is the primary action of any specifically 'antidepressant' drug.

The analgesic effects of non-tricyclic classes of antidepressant are less clear. For example, there is some evidence that fluoxetine (Prozac) is also analgesic in AIDS and some other conditions. However, it is not certain which symptoms the drug is acting on, and whether it is malaise that is being improved, or some other aspect of the MDD syndrome (e.g. anxiety or insomnia) that might be contributing towards a depressed mood. David Healy (1998) has argued that SSRIs may be primarily anxiolytic agents, and some patients diagnosed as suffering from MDD may have significant symptoms of anxiety. It is noteworthy that trials have also shown that benzodiazepines and neuroleptics are more effective than placebo when used as antidepressants, so the ability of a drug to produce significant clinical improvement in depressed patients is not very specific.

Phenelzine, the commonest monoamine oxidase inhibitor, is probably an analgesic rather like the tricyclics, and it also has psychostimulant properties rather like amphetamine. Amphetamine itself is a very powerful analgesic. Amphetamine or some of the other psychostimulants may have a role as antidepressants in carefully selected cases who would be at low risk of addiction and who would not be troubled by the side-effects of these drugs.

Speed of response to antidepressants

It is traditionally maintained that antidepressants take from two to six weeks to have a therapeutic effect, when that 'effect' is measured by global, averaged and mood-based scales such as the Hamilton Rating Scale. According to the above model, the apparently delayed effect of tricyclic antidepressants on mood is due to the fact that the response of mood to analgesia is less specific, slower and more unpredictable than the primary analgesic action on malaise symptoms. In physical medicine it may take some days or weeks for a patient's mood to improve after relief of long-term pain or discomfort, as chronic misery may establish habits of gloomy rumination and an accumulation of sad memories.

The analgesic activity of tricyclics – as for other analgesics – has a rapid onset within hours of reaching an effective dose. It is probable that the first observable effects of tricyclics (i.e. an improvement in physical symptoms) would be detected within hours of reaching an effective dose. It is also possible that the drugs are effective in lower doses than are usually given in psychiatric practice. General practitioners who are treating mild depression often obtain excellent results with lower doses than are considered to be effective in the more severe cases seen in psychiatric practice. Probably this is a dose effect, with severe malaise requiring a higher dose to control it.

However, due to the long half-life of many tricyclics, and also the problem of getting used to side-effects, it is often the case that doses of tricyclics must be escalated slowly. This means that an effective therapeutic blood level of drug may not be reached for several days or even several weeks. However, this is not a slow *onset* of drug action – it is merely a delay in reaching therapeutic blood levels.

Following prolonged malaise, the accumulation of dysphoric memories might alter a person's habitual cognitive style (i.e. their mood). This means that even when they have obtained relief from the current state of malaise, their mood will not immediately improve, and it may not improve at all. This is quite frequently observed – for example, in patients who 'objectively' have greatly improved with regard to their level of activity, appetite, sleep, etc., as a result of antidepressant treatment, but who still feel sad. The antidepressants have 'worked' in the sense that they have alleviated the symptoms which they are effective in treating, but the patient's mood has not improved.

This happens because sadness has many causes in addition to malaise. Misery can be caused by anxiety, emotional blunting, motor side-effects such as akathesia, and indeed by any sustained aversive state. Moreover, even when they are effective, antidepressants cannot transform a whole life and personality – at best they can only alleviate certain symptoms. By concentrating on measuring *mood* as an index of drug effectiveness, researchers on the mode of action of antidepressants have been studying the wrong outcome variable. This is almost as misguided as it would be to measure the effectiveness of aspirin by asking someone how happy they are, rather than asking them whether their headache has improved.

There is an urgent need for new and valid measurement scales to measure the severity of sickness behaviour in order to evaluate the effectiveness of antidepressants. A specifically active antidepressant should have a significant effect on the core symptoms of malaise within hours of reaching an effective dose. Mood is a different matter, and may take several weeks to lift, or it may not lift at all if chronic low mood has had a long-term effect on the person- ality or if a person's life circumstances are so miserable that they make sadness an inevitable response.

This prediction that effective antidepressant activity depends upon an analgesic action with rapid onset has important therapeutic implications. Current practice looks for lifting of mood as evidence of effectiveness and (correctly) assumes that it usually takes four to six weeks for mood to respond to antidepressants. This has been inter- preted as meaning that the doctor should wait for a couple of months before trying another drug.

However, this is probably the wrong approach. Antide- pressants work on malaise, not on mood. Therefore clinical attention should focus on malaise symptoms, not on mood, and a very rapid improvement in symptoms of malaise would be expected as soon as an active drug level is reached. If there is no improvement in malaise symptoms, then another drug should be tried without delay.

If therapeutic trials could be shortened to a week at a therapeutic dose, or even shorter, it would mean that the 'trial-and-error' process of discovering an effective antide- pressant would be much more rapid. Assuming that this strategy could enable much swifter identification of an effec- tive therapeutic agent for each specific patient, then it might represent a major breakthrough in the treatment of depression.

The enormous length of time taken in current practice to conclude that a drug has *not* worked means that many patients will get better spontaneously during this period. This is especially the case in view of the fact that patients will usually be depressed for several weeks or months before they even see a psychiatrist, and most episodes of depression resolve without treatment after approximately six months. Many of the apparently 'late responses' to antidepressant treatment may therefore be natural remissions unrelated to the drug, or due to non-specific factors such as the drug improving sleep and appetite.

Clearly, these ideas need formal testing before they can be adopted, but unless antidepressants are pharmacologically different from any other kind of drug that I know of, they *must* act sooner than six weeks after the start of treatment, even if their full effects take longer to become evident. The task is to devise a rating scale that detects the *first signs* of therapeutic response, rather than relying on 'global' scales (such as the Hamilton scale) which do not focus on core symptoms but add up all of the aspects of depression into a single measure.

Clinicians need to recognise that mood is only indirectly related to drug effects. Enquiring about a patient's state of happiness is not a satisfactory way of establishing whether or not an antidepressant drug has worked. We need to know about the specific drug effect on symptoms of malaise.

Future research into depression and antidepressants

One consequence of the malaise theory is that prescribing of treatments for patients with MDD might be done on a more rational basis. Since MDD is a syndrome and not a disease state, and antidepressants are symptomatic treatments rather than disease-modifying agents, it makes sense to treat 'depression' in an explicitly symptomatic fashion.

At present it is usual to prescribe 'an antidepressant' for the diagnosis of 'major depressive disorder' in a black-box and categorical fashion. The drug is matched to the diagnosis, and the choice of drug depends on secondary factors such as side-effects or cost. Instead, specific symptoms could be targeted by specific drugs which influence these particular symptoms. For instance, malaise might be treated with analgesics, trying out several different ones until something effective was found to relieve the aversive feelings.

In patients with malaise and weight loss, tricyclics might be tried, and the choice of tricyclic made on the grounds of whether or not sedation was desirable. Malaise with over-eating and weight gain might be treated with phenelzine, or possibly with a psychostimulant such as amphetamine, pemoline or methylphenidate (Ritalin). Patients who are miserable without malaise, and whose main complaint is of anxiety, might be treated with anxiolytic agents such as selective serotonin reuptake inhibitors (SSRIs), and again the choice of drug could be made on the grounds of whether stimulation or sedation was required.

Anxious patients might benefit from benzodiazepines, if their potential for addiction is low. Sleeplessness could be treated with hypnotics, and more work needs to be done on the quality of sleep that hypnotics provide (it has been suggested that the 'atypical' neuroleptics such as risperi-done and olanzepine may provide a better quality of sleep than the traditional sleeping tablets such as lorazepam). Psychotic symptoms such as bizarre delusions and halluci-nations could be treated with antidelirium therapy such as ECT or hypnotics. Agitated behaviour driven by extreme emotions could be treated with neuroleptics. Of course, caution would need to be exercised over drug interactions, but this way of tailoring treatments to a specific patient's symptoms has greater therapeutic potential than the simplistic notion of categorical prescribing for categorical diagnosis. Instead, the aim is not to treat the syndrome of depression, but rather to try to break down the syndrome into symptoms, and tailor the treatment to the symptom profile of each individual patient.

As a long-term goal, it might be a reasonable strategy in treating the syndrome of MDD to seek *disease-modifying* agents, which operate to normalise either the primary cause of sickness behaviour or the cytokines which mediate that sickness behaviour. In this context it might be fruitful to explore the use of anti-inflammatory drugs in MDD (e.g. very-low-dose glucocorticoids, which have recently been found to be effective in the treatment of rheumatoid arthritis and chronic fatigue).

Analgesics as antidepressants

As tricyclic antidepressants are analgesic, and this is assumed to explain their therapeutic action, it would be predicted that 'traditional' analgesics should also be effective as antidepressants. It is an intriguing possibility that traditional analgesics such as paracetamol, aspirin or the non-steroidal anti-inflammatory drugs (NSAIDs) might also be effective against the symptom of malaise which is at the core of depression. Indeed, it is an open question whether or not much of the self-medication with simple analgesics that goes on may actually be done for the purposes of mood manipulation rather than pain relief. Certainly the belief that aspirin 'picks you up when you are down' is common enough.

My suggestion is that antidepressants should be targeted specifically at malaise symptoms. The prospects for drug development are intriguing. Tricyclics are not remarkable for their effectiveness as antidepressants (at least as currently prescribed). They also have unpleasant and sometimes dangerous side-effects. There is certainly great scope for improvement of antidepressants.

It is quite possible that more specific and effective and less toxic antidepressants could be engineered or discovered if the process was informed by increased precision in defining the nature of the target symptom of malaise, and if there was an improved understanding of the desired pharmacological effect in alleviating malaise.

Centrally acting analgesics of the opiate class should probably have a role in the management of MDD when malaise symptoms are dominant. Before the advent of ECT and the discovery of tricyclics, opium was considered by many authorities to be the best and most specific treatment for 'melancholia'. In the 1970s, when the endogenous opiates (enkephalins and endorphins) were discovered, there was a resurgence of interest in this possibility. Several studies were published which suggested a useful therapeutic role for opiates in depression. However, the results were somewhat confusing, and the field seems to have been abandoned without the questions ever being properly resolved.

It seems highly likely that opiates would be effective anti-malaise analgesics, and hence effective antidepressants. Certainly opiates such as codeine are commonly used and effective in improving symptoms of colds and flu, which suggests that the same would probably be true with regard to MDD. At least opiates would be worth trying in malaise-dominated depressed patients who are unresponsive to, or unable to tolerate, more conventional antidepressants.

Formal studies would be needed to determine the potential usefulness of opiates in the treatment of subgroups of MDD patients. Interestingly, there are no reports of addiction when opiates are used in depression, but even if there were to be a small risk, this may be justifiable on the grounds of relieving suffering and improving social functioning. However, it is generally believed that when opiates are used appropriately *as analgesics*, dependence is very unlikely to become a problem.

Conversely, if antidepressants are analgesic for malaise, perhaps the usage of tricyclics could be expanded more widely into the treatment of other physical illnesses typified by malaise. For instance, tricyclics might be effective agents for the symptomatic treatment of acute infections, and inflammatory, neoplastic or other types of immune activation. Perhaps tricyclics may even have a role in the management of colds and flu.

Action of SSRIs – emotion buffering?

The class of drugs known as selective serotonin reuptake inhibitors (SSRIs), such as fluoxetine (Prozac) and paroxetine (Seroxat), constitute the other major class of 'antidepressants' apart from the tricyclics. Yet SSRIs are probably not analgesic, or at least their effect as analgesics appears to be much weaker than that of the tricyclics. However, they

are very effective psychotropic drugs in that they have transformed the lives of many patients for the better.

David Healy (1997) has suggested that SSRIs function
mainly as anxiolytics. This is certainly consistent with the
fact that in clinical practice SSRIs have largely replaced the
benzodiazepines in the treatment of anxiety symptoms and
anxiety-dominated syndromes. However, their psychological
action seems to be very different to that of the benzodiazepines. The most striking therapeutic effect of SSRIs could be
described as *emotion-buffering*.

Emotion-buffering (when it happens, and it does not
happen in all patients) is usually experienced as a pleasant
feeling of a 'safety net' under one's emotions, preventing
large and unpleasant downswings. Bad things happen, and
people still feel bad about them, but *not as bad* as they do
when not taking SSRIs. Moment-to-moment emotions
probably do not change at all. For most of the time, people
feel the same when they are taking SSRIs as they do when
they are not taking the drug. However, although everyday
emotions may be unaffected, the drug gives people a feeling
of confidence that they will not be overwhelmed by negative
feelings.

The flip side to this is that emotion-buffering seems to
work on upswings as well, and patients taking SSRIs often
report that they are not so able to feel 'high' or ecstatic as
they used to. Some people find this unpleasant and cannot
tolerate the drug, while others do not seem to mind this
effect, or think that it is more than compensated for by the
prevention of downswings. A lot depends on personal
constitution.

If it is agreed that emotion-buffering is the primary useful
action of SSRIs, then it may be worth speculating how this
might occur. Since emotions are the brain's registration of
body states, my suggestion is that SSRIs work on the body.
Rapid changes in body states are mainly controlled by the
autonomic (sympathetic and parasympathetic) nervous
system, which controls the blood vessels and internal
organs. Perhaps SSRIs act by stabilising the autonomic
nervous system in order to damp down the powerful and
sometimes 'overwhelming' activation of the nervous system.

For instance, if you get involved in an unpleasant row, this activates the sympathetic nervous system and may provoke a rapid and massive release of adrenaline and noradrenaline. If something happens that disgusts you, it may provoke a similar surge in acetylcholine that stimulates the gut. My suggestion is that SSRIs act upon the autonomic system to damp down these large-scale activations of the autonomic nervous system, thus avoiding extremes of emotion without affecting everyday fluctuations. SSRIs are not so much anti-malaise analgesics as anti-extreme-emotion agents.

Summary – the nature of depression

It has been argued that major depressive disorder is inappropriate sickness behaviour, that the syndrome of MDD is generated by abnormalities in cytokines, and that antidepressants exert their specifically beneficial effects through analgesic action on the core dysphoric emotion of malaise.

The malaise theory does not, of course, simply replace current ideas about the nature of depression and the mode of action of antidepressants. There is a considerable measure of redefinition as well as redescription. Not everyone diagnosed as suffering from MDD would have sickness behaviour or be characterised by malaise, and not everyone with malaise would be diagnosable as having MDD. In particular, I would expect that many patients with milder forms of MDD are mainly suffering from anxiety and mood swings, which is why SSRIs are so often useful. Not all current 'antidepressants' will be analgesics, and not all analgesics will be anti-malaise antidepressants.

Therefore, what I am doing is carving out a new and coherent diagnostic syndrome from the heterogeneous mass that is 'depression', and suggesting the target symptoms against which drug effectiveness can be evaluated.

It will also be noticed that I have not compared the malaise theory with existing theories about depression and antidepressant action. This is mainly because the malaise theory operates at a quite different level of explanation from the dominant group of theories which are more or less based on the 'amine hypothesis'. The malaise theory describes psychological abnormalities associated with a pathological somatic immune state, and the effects of drugs in terms of their action on symptoms. By contrast, the amine hypothesis describes neurotransmitter abnormalities and neurotransmitter-level pharmacological effects as they apply to syndromal diagnoses. It is still too early to say whether or not these two types of theory can ultimately be synthesised, but if they are both true, then ultimately they can be integrated.

Mood management and self-help

As well as being – I hope – true, the malaise theory of depression seems to be a clearer, more comprehensible and clinically useful model of depression than the current mainstream model. And given that depression is so common, the management of this disorder cannot be wholly a matter for professionals and experts. There is an important role for self-diagnosis, self-treatment and the self-evaluation of this treatment.

When a person complains of 'sadness' or perceives that they are sad, the first step is to establish the nature of this sadness, as there are innumerable ways of feeling sad. If the sadness seems to be based upon malaise, then the symptoms of malaise – and not the sadness – become the focus of physical treatment. Whatever treatments are tried, from simple analgesics through to the formal 'antidepressants', it then makes sense to monitor treatment by the effect on malaise.

This style of self-monitoring is a skill which requires practice, and some people seem to lack the ability altogether. What is needed is the ability to look behind the statement 'I feel awful', and pinpoint as precisely as possible what it is that feels awful and how. This allows a more helpful focus than is sometimes adopted. For instance, many people respond to the 'I feel awful' feeling of malaise ('like a black cloud pressing on my head') by getting intoxi-cated and obliterating consciousness to a greater or lesser degree. Therefore people may get drunk or drugged, or take anxiolytics so that they feel 'doped' but suffer less. A better strategy may be to leave consciousness intact, but to remove the feeling of malaise (i.e. to disperse the black cloud).

However, even if it is effective, removal of malaise does not produce feelings of happiness or gratification (except for the short-term sense of relief at gaining ease from suffering – the best thing about hitting your head against a brick wall is that it is lovely when you stop). Removal of malaise potentially allows people to enjoy themselves, and it allows the body to enact gratifying emotions once again, but this does not *ensure* that such gratifying emotions will in fact be enacted. Sometimes people are disappointed that antidepres-sants have not made them happy, and interpret this as meaning that the drugs have not worked. That is expecting too much.

If you have flu and are miserable, exhausted and have a 'black cloud' pressing on your head, then when you eventually recover from the flu (or take effective sympto-matic treatment), this does not mean that you will automa-tically become happy. In fact, it may be difficult to become happy if you have been living in a dysphoric state for several weeks – you may have developed habits of gloomy interpretation and stocked your memory with gloomy thoughts. It still requires the usual effort of life to seek grati-fication, and this is seldom an easy matter, especially when one is debilitated by illness. However, it should certainly be *easier* to experience pleasure if you are rid of that black cloud.

And that, more or less, is the modest yet extremely worthwhile contribution of antidepressants to the human condition.

CHAPTER TEN

Mania

Mania is the least well known of the serious psychiatric illnesses. The nearest common equivalent is the word 'maniac' when used to describe someone who is violently out of control. The nearest a normal person gets to experiencing mania is probably after certain kinds of jet lag or after staying up all night – that buoyed-up feeling of being full of energy and immune to tiredness with no need to relax or sleep (and getting very irritable with anyone who tries to suggests that you need to take a break). Mania is one of the most difficult illnesses to explain, not least because the patient usually denies that he or she is ill, and may indeed feel abnormally healthy.

Under traditional diagnostic schemes, mania is regarded as an *affective* disorder – that is, an illness of the mood and the opposite of depression. Whereas depression is a low, miserable mood, mania is often a high, elated, grandiose mood. There are two kinds of mania, namely hypomania, which is milder and non-psychotic, and mania, which is the full-blown syndrome including hallucinations, delusions, and rapid speech characterised by frequent changes of subject.

Manic people are overactive, rushing around continually without taking a break. They talk fast, too much and too loudly, hardly sleep, and are short-tempered and often aggressive. Full-blown mania is usually characterised by a wild over-confidence and over-estimation of one's ability, often combined with a paranoid belief that these abilities are being thwarted by other people who happen to be around.

Energy, confidence and activity in the absence of

hypomania are valuable attributes, which probably explains why the tendency to mania persists in the population, and why genes associated with mania have not been eliminated from the population. So long as actual mania does not emerge, then a somewhat 'manic' (i.e. energetic, confident and fatigue-resistant) temperament is often an asset – at least in some jobs, such as sales and politics. The question is, what pushes such a person over into the damaging and maladaptive state of mania?

Problems with current concepts

Being manic or 'high' does not seem to be an illness in the same way as depression. Of course, when mania is psychotic, and so severe as to result in jumbled speech, bizarre delusions (e.g. that the manic person is Napoleon, Jesus Christ or God himself) and hallucinations, then there is no problem in any objective observer conceiving it as an illness – the patient appears to be 'raving mad'. However, the more common state of *hypo*mania can be very difficult to diagnose.

Yet hypomania is potentially a very serious condition precisely because neither the sufferers nor their family and friends recognise that it is an illness. Someone who is 'high' undergoes a change in personality which may destroy their life. They may quarrel with their spouse and break up a marriage; they may quarrel with their boss, be sacked and become unemployed; they may spend money until they are deep in debt, and behave with dangerous irresponsibility – driving recklessly, getting into fights, or having promiscuous and unprotected sex. Despite the high self-confidence, this mood is brittle and impulsive, and there is a considerable risk of suicide. The social devastation wreaked by mania may be at least as great as that caused by any other psychiatric illness.

The nature of mania remains obscure. The idea that it is a *mood* disorder stems from Kraepelin's suggestion some 100 years ago. However, as I have argued earlier for depression, mood is not a primary biological variable, but instead we should regard mood as the *outcome* of other biological variables. Mood is merely shorthand for certain characteristic modes of behaviour.

In any case, the mood in mania is not very specific, being extremely variable and changeable. There is even a 'dysphoric' mania recognised which is characterised by a low and unhappy mood (i.e. a 'depressed' mood), but combined with a typical manic pattern of overactivity, over-talkativeness and a therapeutic responsivity to antimanic treatments.

So if mania is not a mood disorder, then what is it?

Arousal and analgesia

I suggest that there are two core components to the syndrome of hypomania, namely excessive arousal and analgesia. Full-blown mania arises when chronic, severe sleep deprivation is added to the picture of hypomania. Sleep deprivation creates a delirious, functionally brain-impaired state which leads to psychotic symptoms such as jumbled speech, hallucinations and delusions.

First I shall consider excessive arousal. Arousal is a very general psychological term, which refers to the continuum of alertness – a continuum that ranges from lack of envir-onmental awareness, coma and sleep at one end to states of high vigilance, energy and activity at the other end.

Most people are familiar with the experience of periods of time during which they feel highly aroused – wide awake, driven, unable to stop working or talking, and overbearing in manner. Sometimes, paradoxically, hyperarousal can occur when we are in fact over-tired – for example, after a sleepless night or a long journey. These are times when we are paradoxically flooded by energy and unable (or unwilling) to switch off and relax. For example, I recently missed a night's sleep when flying back to England from the USA. When I got home I felt utterly drained, but found it difficult to sit down and rest, and impossible to sleep.

Habitual levels of arousal vary widely between indivi-duals, and this is one of the most obvious and important aspects of temperament. Some people have more energy than others, get tired less easily, and need less sleep. They may live in a state close to hypomania for long periods of time. Perhaps it is more common to experience periods of energy alternating with periods of passivity, withdrawal and rest – this is the so-called *cyclothymic* temperament.

I suggest that the aroused state in its most extreme form is one component of mania, and is about as close as most of us get to mania. What stops this going further and ending up as pathological mania is the negative feedback of *fatigue*. When we are overactive, eventually fatigue catches up with us and we stop, rest and sleep. The biochemical basis of fatigue is probably related to the same complex group of immune chemicals that we encountered in the chapter on depression, namely the cytokines. A build-up of cytokines and other similar substances is probably what slows us down and forces us to rest. Fatigue is an example of 'negative feedback' in which biological systems balance themselves. Too much activity leads to fatigue, which allows us to recharge our energy supplies to enable more activity subsequently.

So although fatigue is a subjectively unpleasant feeling, like pain, it is also a vital biological adaptation, again like pain. Without fatigue we might carry on and on charging around and doing things until we collapsed and died of exhaustion. That is exactly what used to happen to some manic patients in the days before powerful sedative and tranquillising drugs were available. 'Raging maniacs' would charge around the locked wards for day after day, never resting, never sleeping, until they collapsed and died, usually of heart failure. Acute, severe mania was a fatal illness.

It can be seen that removal of the subjectively aversive sensation that is fatigue can be dangerous because it allows activity to continue when it ought to stop. Since fatigue is an aversive, unpleasant sensation, it seems reasonable to suggest that fatigue can in fact be regarded as *a form of pain*. Substances that remove aversive sensations of pain are called analgesics, and I suggest that these same substances may also remove the aversive sensations we term fatigue – sensations that are akin to pain and which may share similar biochemical causes.

The reason why some people become overactive in the first place may be a matter of temperament or personality. It is well known that people who suffer from the illness of mania are also usually individuals who tend to be energetic, confident and highly active even when they are not ill. Energy, confidence and activity are valuable attributes so long as actual mania does not emerge. However, such a person may have been forced to ignore fatigue and remain active for some reason beyond their control (e.g. due to demands of work, travel or family life). They may stay up late, or stay up all night. In a susceptible person this stress could act to initiate the self-sustaining state that we call hypomania or mania.

My hypothesis is that the factor which probably switches temperamentally hyperactive people over into hypomania is the production of some endogenous, internally produced anti-fatigue analgesic substance (or, alternatively, perhaps taking some drug with anti-fatigue analgesic properties).

I suggest that mania is characterised by the inappropriate production of some kind of endogenous analgesic that prevents fatigue and allows the manic patient to continue with hyperactivity without experiencing the negative feedback of fatigue. When an over-aroused state is combined with an analgesic that removes fatigue, then hypomania occurs. This is a state in which overactivity is no longer held in check by fatigue.

Endogenous opiates as anti-fatigue analgesics in mania

For overarousal to tip over into hypomania, the normal sensation of fatigue needs to be suppressed or overridden by an analgesic agent. The human body produces its own analgesics of various kinds. The 'high' mood of mania is a secondary consequence of the ability to remain active without fatigue. Such an ability usually makes people feel good, powerful and impressed with themselves. The analgesic activity means that there is a loss of perception of many of the negative feelings that accompany normal life – a blunting of the sense of shame, shyness and fear.

If mania is caused by the inappropriate activity of some kind of endogenous analgesic that prevents fatigue, the question arises as to what this analgesic might be. An analgesic drug could be responsible – for example, amphetamine, which produces a state very similar to mania. However, as many patients with manic symptoms are not taking any drugs, this strongly suggests that there is an *endogenous* or internally produced analgesic substance which abolishes fatigue in the manic patient.

The nature of this endogenous, anti-fatigue analgesic is not known, but it is reasonable to speculate about its identity. Perhaps the most obvious candidates for an endogenous analgesic that could allow hyperactivity to develop into hypomania are the *endogenous opiates* (e.g. the endorphins and enkephalins). The best understood of the endorphins is beta-endorphin, which is a peptide hormone (i.e. a short protein molecule) that circulates in the blood. Beta-endorphin is secreted from the anterior pituitary gland and is derived from the same precursor molecule as the 'stress hormone' ACTH (which causes the secretion of the steroid hormone cortisol), and beta-endorphin is also released under conditions of stress, pain, physical activity and probably fatigue. It is termed an 'endogenous opiate' because it has the same type of pharmacological effect as the opiates such as morphine, heroin, pethidine and codeine, which all act on the same general class of hormone receptors.

If there was excessive secretion of endogenous opiates such as beta-endorphin, then this could be at least partly responsible for precipitating mania. The possibility that this occurs is suggested by the observation that 'exogenous' opiates given as drugs have the same ability to induce mania. There are numerous papers in the literature which suggest that opiate drugs may precipitate mania in susceptible individuals. This effect may be surprising, given that opiates are sedative, and it adds support to the theory that the analgesic effect is a vital component of mania.

The arousal–analgesia model for hypomania leading on to full mania

We can now suggest a plausible sequence of events that leads to hypomania. In the first place, there must be a hyper-aroused, *driven* state leading to overactivity. Perhaps a young businessman is trying to achieve an almost impossible deadline and stays up night after night completing paperwork. At first he feels exhausted, but he keeps pushing himself and then finds that the more he does, the less tired he feels.

Normally, overactivity would be stopped by negative feedback from fatigue. However, if hyper-secretion of endogenous opiates occurs, these may have an analgesic effect that removes the negative feedback of fatigue. In the businessman's body great floods of endorphins lead to immunity to tiredness, and a feeling of invulnerability. The businessman starts to feel that he is breaking through to a new level of ability – after all, he can work twice as long as anyone else, he feels fine, his mind is sharp, and the work he produces is great! He has no time for the slow, dull plodders (such as his wife) who tell him he needs a break, a rest or a sleep – *they* may need it, but he does not. He is clearly superior. He asks his wife to run a bath for him – this seems to take forever, and then when he gets in the water is too cold! The businessman turns on his wife, and sees that she and his children are cowering in the corner as if he was some kind of wild animal. Disgusted at their feebleness, he storms out of the house slamming the door. Perhaps he should go and find a prostitute instead of his wife – after all, a man of his energy cannot expect to be satisfied by just one woman...

Chronic, severe sleep deprivation as the cause of manic psychotic symptoms

Hyperactivity continues, which provides the 'stress' necessary to stimulate further endorphin secretion. Overactivity is accompanied by diminished sleep. If overactivity is so severe as to reduce sleep below the minimum amount necessary for human health (usually about four hours a night) and for several days in a row, then the patient might become delirious due to sleep deprivation. The delirium will lead to classic 'psychotic' symptoms such as hallucinations, bizarre delusions and jumbled speech ('thought disorder') superimposed on non-fatiguing hypomanic overactivity.

Thus the full state of mania might emerge, with overactivity, lack of fatigue, and psychotic symptoms. The businessman leaves his desk, roams the streets trying to enlist people for his new project, telephones colleagues all through the night, takes a plane to the central office (no time to waste!), harangues the chief executive for his failure to allocate resources to the new project, and gets kicked out of headquarters. He realises that the company are all in a conspiracy to hold back his new ideas. He has stopped sleeping, although he isn't really fully awake, but in a fluctuating twilight state, finding it difficult to concentrate or frame his thoughts.

He begins to hear voices, probably mobile-telephone messages in which the chief executive is instructing a gang to find and kill him (although no one else seems to hear these voices). He tries to inform the police about the whole thing, but they just look blank and too stupid to understand, even when he shouts and shakes the desk sergeant to try to get some sense into him. The next thing he knows, the hard working businessman finds himself in a psychiatric ward – probably (as he imagines) on the orders of the chief executive. . .

Recovery – mania terminated by deep sleep

At a certain point mania can become self-sustaining. Sleep deprivation, once established, might itself be sufficient 'stress' to maintain the hyper-secretion of endogenous analgesics, which would sustain the sleep deprivation. Even if the initial provoking incident was removed, the manic state might then continue until the positive-feedback cycle of sleep deprivation and endogenous anti-fatigue analgesia was broken. The cycle might be broken by sleep, as fatigue eventually took hold.

After the businessman arrives on the ward he is given a tablet 'to help him sleep'. Reluctantly he takes it and blacks out for hours. When he wakens his head is much clearer, although he cannot really remember how he ended up in a psychiatric hospital. Over the next few days he begins to feel calmer, and his incredible self-confidence is invaded by doubts, embarrassment and despair as he discovers that he has been given the sack.

There is a self-sustaining cycle of overactivity that causes endorphin hyper-secretion, which abolishes fatigue, which in turn allows more overactivity. Once this positive-feedback cycle has been terminated by deep sleep, then manic symptoms may resolve rapidly and completely. If the cycle is not broken, the mania may persist for weeks or months. However, quick and total recovery from even very severe and prolonged mania is quite usual, although even fully recovered people seldom fully acknowledge that they were ill at the time of mania. After all, they felt so well, so confident, so full of energy...

This arousal–analgesia model predicts that full-blown mania is a delirious state. If this is so, the symptoms of delirium would be present, and an electroencephalogram (EEG) would be abnormal (if it proves possible to record one on a manic patient). An EEG abnormality would be defined as a recording that is abnormal compared to the patient's own non-manic EEG, so later, post-recovery EEGs are required for comparison with the 'manic' EEG. There are many similarities between mania and 'agitated delirium', poor concentration and distractibility being particularly prominent in both conditions. I suggest that the two conditions cannot be clearly distinguished and are indeed different aspects of the same spectrum. The difference between agitated delirium and mania probably lies in the cause and long-term prognosis rather than in the cross-sectional psychopathology.

I suggest that full-blown mania with psychotic symptoms caused by delirium is therefore properly treated by *sleep*. This needs to be deep restorative sleep, which can usually be induced by neuroleptic drugs and sedatives such as lorazepam. Alternatively, mania can be rapidly resolved by one or two treatments with ECT, which (as argued in a previous chapter) may serve as a sleep surrogate or induce a deep sleep in the post-ictal period.

The traditional interpretation

The above sequence of events represents a fairly uncontroversial account of the *events* of a manic episode, but my interpretation of *causes* is highly unconventional. In the first place, sleep deprivation is conventionally regarded as a symptom of mania, not as a cause of it. Manic patients are assumed to be sleepless because of their elevated mood, and the sleeplessness is not given an important role in generating symptoms such as hallucinations and delusions.

Moreover, the effective treatment of mania by neuroleptic drugs is not regarded as being directed at causing sleep. Rather, neuroleptics are viewed as either general-purpose 'behaviour control' drugs, which reduce physical and psychological overactivity, or they are seen as 'antipsychotic' agents which specifically remove symptoms such as delusions and hallucinations. The neuroleptic drugs used to treat mania may not be of the sedative kind, and they are often given at regular intervals throughout the day. By contrast, I would advocate that specifically sedative drugs are used to treat mania, and these sedative agents would be given (if possible) only at night in order to promote the natural sleep-waking cycle, and to avoid daytime somnolence (which may also make it more difficult to sleep at the proper time).

In addition, ECT is very seldom given for mania except as a last resort, despite an abundance of evidence for its effectiveness. Without ECT, patients may not respond to drugs, and may remain manic for many weeks or months. However, psychiatrists are reluctant to use ECT in mania, probably because it is regarded as an antidepressant treatment, and there seems to be no rationale for using ECT to treat an illness that is perceived to be 'the opposite' of depression.

Altogether, the field of mania is an extremely confused one, and the fundamental problem stems from the classification of mania as a *mood* disorder. Once the syndrome is considered in terms of its symptom profile, then everything becomes much clearer.

Other anti-fatigue endogenous analgesics in mania

Endogenous opiates may not be the only analgesics responsible for mania. There may be other endogenous molecules with anti-fatigue analgesic properties – for example, the glucocorticoid hormones such as cortisol.

Glucocorticoids (e.g. cortisol secreted from the adrenal gland) are analgesic, anti-inflammatory hormones that act upon most of the cells in the body. Compared with endorphins, which act within minutes of secretion, cortisol has a slow onset of action over a period of many hours or several days. (Cortisol exerts its action by diffusing into the cell nucleus and affecting DNA transcription, while endorphin binds to a cell-surface receptor to induce rapid changes in messenger molecules within the cell.) ACTH is the hormone that stimulates cortisol secretion from the adrenal gland, and ACTH is co-secreted together with beta-endorphin in response to stresses such as pain, fear or anger. Thus there is a tendency for cortisol levels to increase together with endorphins – hyper-secretion of one might well be accompanied by hyper-secretion of the other. Cortisol might provide a slower-acting but more powerful and sustained form of anti-fatigue analgesia.

Under normal, adaptive conditions, glucocorticoids may work together with the endorphins to provide useful analgesia which allows a more effective 'fight-or-flight' behaviour. It is well known that under conditions of excitement or danger (e.g. during a battle or a sports contest), there is a temporary insensibility to pain which may be useful for allowing escape. However, the combined analgesia of endorphins and cortisol would be maladaptive when it removes the necessary negative feedback of fatigue.

The role of glucocorticoids in mania is also supported by the psychiatric literature. Many papers have described elevated cortisol levels in patients with mania, and cortisol resistance to dexamethasone suppression (which is also indicative of excess cortisol secretion). Mania is itself a well-established (although uncommon) side-effect of treatment with glucocorticoid drugs such as prednisone or hydrocortisone. For example, I have seen grandiose manic delusions developing in a man who was given steroids for multiple sclerosis, and those symptoms subsided when the steroid dose was reduced. Mania is also sometimes found among patients with Cushing's disease who produce excess ACTH (although Cushing's patients more often feel ill and depressed; perhaps this is due to the catabolic, i.e. tissue-destroying, effects which occur when glucocorticoids are chronically evelated).

Psychopharmacological analgesia increases susceptibility to mania

Further evidence that mania is a consequence of arousal and analgesia comes from psychopharmacology. The best examples of drugs that produce a manic syndrome are the psychostimulant drug amphetamine and its analogues.

It is well known that amphetamine increases arousal, but it is less well known that it is also an extremely powerful analgesic – almost as powerful as morphine. This fact is abundantly documented in the literature, although – probably due to fear of addiction – amphetamine is very seldom used as an analgesic in clinical practice. My suggestion is that the analgesic effect is a major element of the effect that amphetamine has in reducing fatigue (and amphetamine is probably the most effective known agent for reducing fatigue). This combination of increased arousal and analgesia makes amphetamine a potent agent for inducing manic states.

Indeed, any agent that produces arousal and analgesia should be able to cause (or increase the likelihood of developing) a state resembling hypomania. For instance, caffeine is a much weaker drug than amphetamine, but it shares the ability to produce increased arousal with a significant analgesic effect. The alerting effects of caffeine are well known, but its analgesic effect is less well documented, although caffeine is included in many proprietary painkillers. However, according to a recent estimate, caffeine is probably about equivalent in its analgesic effect to paracetamol.

The 'wired' state that results from large-scale ingestion of caffeine could therefore be regarded as a reasonable model for a mild-state hypomania, although the unpleasant side-effects of excess caffeine, and its rather weak analgesic effects, mean that its over-use is not exactly equivalent to hypomania.

Induced fatigue as therapy for mania

The role of anti-fatigue analgesia in causing mania suggests a potential therapeutic avenue with regard to deliberately induced fatigue as a treatment for mania. If hypomania is necessarily accompanied by analgesia for fatigue, then any 'anti-analgesic' intervention which restored the proper feeling of fatigue might act to restore negative feedback, and therefore be potentially effective in terminating mania.

There is little evidence on this matter, but we might speculate and make a few suggestions as to how this could be achieved. The best-known anti-analgesic is naloxone, which is an antagonist to morphine and some other opiates, including endorphins. There is suggestive (although inconclusive) evidence in the literature that naloxone, when given in sufficient doses, has antimanic properties. The therapeutic effectiveness of naloxone in mania would certainly make sense in those patients whose mania was considered to have been induced by the anti-fatigue analgesic effects of endogenous opiates.

The main class of substances that cause fatigue includes the cytokines. It has already been argued that cytokines cause the syndrome of major depressive disorder in which fatigue and other painful and dysphoric feelings are so prominent. Some cytokines are 'hyperalgesic' – that is, they lower the threshold for pain and also for fatigue. This implies that an infusion of cytokines (e.g. interferon) might be a very effective way of terminating a manic attack. The side-effects of cytokine infusion would undoubtedly be unpleasant, just as they are when interferon is used to treat cancer or viral illnesses. None the less, cytokine treatment of mania may be a viable option in extreme or resistant cases.

One way of testing this prediction of the efficacy of cytokine therapy would be to find out whether mania can be 'spontaneously' terminated by a cytokine-inducing illness, such as influenza (which typically produces profound fatigue and exhaustion of a kind which is incompatible with mania). Observational studies might be able to answer such a question.

However, for the present, the main treatment for acute mania is with the class of drugs known as the neuroleptics, and it is to the action of this group of drugs that we shall now turn.

CHAPTER ELEVEN

Neuroleptics

The current first-line treatment of an *acute* episode of hypomania or mania, or indeed an acute psychosis of any kind, is with the neuroleptic class of drugs. Neuroleptics are also known as 'antipsychotics' and 'major tranquillisers', and they include drugs such as chlorpromazine (Largactil), haloperidol (Haldol), long-acting injections such as Modecate and Depixol, and more recent 'atypical neuroleptic' agents such clozepine (Clozaril).

Chlorpromazine is regarded as one of the most successful drugs in the history of medicine, and it broke upon psychiatry with such force that the subject was completely transformed. Neuroleptic drugs revolutionised the treatment of schizophrenia and other severe psychiatric illnesses. Indeed, chlorpromazine is sometimes credited with having 'emptied the mental hospitals' in the 1950s and 1960s, by enabling many chronically psychotic patients to live in the community.

However, like most of the other classes of psychiatric drugs, there is no generally accepted understanding about what neuroleptics actually *do*. It is known that they shorten episodes of illness and reduce the relapse rate, but how they do this remains unclear.

In my view, neuroleptics are essentially drugs that *blunt emotion*, in the sense that they blunt the enactment of emotions. In other words, neuroleptics block the ability to produce body states that correspond to emotions, so these drugs diminish anxiety, rendering the viscera unresponsive, in a sense by 'fixing' the muscles rather than by relaxing them (as diazepam does). The name 'neuroleptic' actually means something that 'seizes' the nervous system, and this term communicates well the idea that neuroleptics 'hold' the body and make it less responsive to the autonomic nervous system and hormones, thereby preventing the physical enactment of large emotional changes – whether pleasurable or aversive.

In high doses, some neuroleptics act as 'chemical strait-jackets', having a tendency to immobilise patients. This is not the case for all neuroleptics, and the dose at which the effect becomes apparent varies between individuals (perhaps at a dose roughly ten times that for the neuroleptic effect). This 'strait-jacketing' may be a short-term necessity for severely violent patients (or at least it may be the best available option among a variety of unpleasant alternatives such as physical restraint).

Mode of action of neuroleptics

Although their chemistry and molecular pharmacology have been the subject of vast amounts of research, the mode of action of neuroleptics is not known. Many people regard them as 'antipsychotic' agents, and assume that their therapeutic effect is simply to remove abnormal psychological events such as hallucinations and delusions while leaving the rest of cognition intact and unaffected.

However, closer study has revealed that neuroleptics probably do *not* remove psychotic symptoms (at least, not in chronically psychotic patients), but rather they reduce the unpleasant emotional impact of hallucinations or delusions, so that patients become 'indifferent' to them, ignore them, and cease to act upon them. As one patient said: 'Oh yes, the voices are still there, I just don't listen to them anymore.'

However, it seems more plausible that neuroleptics are drugs that act primarily upon movement, and that the therapeutic effect is actually a milder version of the 'immobilisation' or chemical strait-jacket produced by high-dose neuroleptics. Immobilisation of muscles prevents emotional expression, and blunted expression actually blunts emotional perception.

Side-effects or therapeutic effects?

The most notorious side-effect of the neuroleptic drugs is their action on muscles – the 'motor' side-effects. I suggest that the motor effects of neuroleptics are in fact also the cause of the therapeutic effect of emotional blunting.

Neuroleptics produce a wide range of movement disorders, some of which are short-lasting, while others may be permanent. The most typical effects are Parkinsonian (i.e. like Parkinson's disease), so the triad of muscular rigidity, tremor and bradykinesia (difficulty in initiating movement) is common. A motor side-effect that is more difficult to describe is 'akathesia', which is a very unpleasant sense of motor restlessness, an inability to become comfortable. Neuroleptics can produce contortions and twisting – for example, a forced upward gaze of the eyes (oculogyric crisis). Some effects may be long-lasting or even permanent – a syndrome that is termed tardive dyskinesia. This usually consists of facial movements such as chewing of the jaw, pouting of the lips and protrusion of the tongue. Even without such obvious changes, people taking neuroleptics often look subtly different, and have a somewhat blank, staring and 'expressionless' facial appearance.

These motor effects are generally considered to be 'side-effects' and distinct from the therapeutic neuroleptic effect. The recent development of 'atypical' neuroleptics with far fewer and milder motor effects is evidence of this – as atypical neuroleptics are supposed to produce the same therapeutic benefits as the old drugs but without the motor side-effects.

However, in terms of the specifically neuroleptic effect, namely its ability to control disturbed behaviour, the potency of a neuroleptic drug is correlated with its tendency to produce motor side-effects. Thus the most potent drugs used in psychiatric emergencies to control violent patients, namely drugs such as haloperidol and droperidol, are also the drugs that are most likely to produce motor side-effects. The 'atypicals' and other neuroleptics that are largely free of motor effects, such as olanzepine or thioridazine, are seldom used to control acutely disturbed behaviour (except in so far as their sedative effects may have an independent and useful role).

Action on the basal ganglia

My suggestion is that the specifically neuroleptic effect is a direct consequence of action on the basal ganglia. The basal ganglia are brain centres that fine-tune movement, and neuroleptics probably act to impair (usually reversibly) the action of these centres. Given the current understanding of emotion as being the brain representation of body changes, it seems plausible to suggest that the emotional blunting which may be therapeutic in some patients on neuroleptics is a consequence of muscle rigidity and other forms of impaired muscle responsivity.

Thus the emotional blunting which is the core psychological effect of neuroleptics is caused by increased muscle rigidity and reduced responsivity of muscles to the autonomic nervous system (such rigidity might be expected to be detectable by electromyelogram). This implies that that the blank face characteristic of a patient on neuroleptics is itself partly responsible for a blunting of emotion, as the brain monitors facial expression as part of its monitoring of emotion.

Feedback from the muscles of facial expression is known to be a factor in perceived emotion – for example, manipulating the face into the shape of a smile actually makes people happier! Similarly, the diminution of facial expression reduces the changes in feedback to the brain and produces a feeling of emotional unresponsivity. Emotional blunting may be unpleasant for someone who is not ill, but blunting may be very welcome to a person who is tormented by delusions and hallucinations.

Since emotions depend on feedback from physical changes in the body, any drug which stiffens (or paralyses) muscles would be expected to reduce or abolish the intensity of emotions that are dependent on enactment in those muscles. Anything which diminishes the physical expression of emotion will also diminish the perception of that emotion in the brain. For instance, patients with spinal cord transection have diminished feedback from the lower body muscles and viscera, and these patients also have diminished intensity of emotions.

Thus emotions are blunted by neuroleptics, and the stronger the motor 'side-effects' of a drug, the more powerful its neuroleptic effect will be. By this account, the 'chemical strait-jacket' effect of high doses of high-potency neuroleptics is merely a more extreme version of the calming effect of low doses of lower-potency neuroleptic drugs. It is not so much a matter of neuroleptic drugs having therapeutic neuroleptic effects and 'Parkinsonian' side-effects, but that these are points on a continuum of action on the basal ganglia. Crudely speaking, the higher the dose, the greater the degree of immobilisation.

Neuroleptics and the somatic marker mechanism

The way in which neuroleptics produce 'indifference' and demotivation can be interpreted in terms of the somatic marker mechanism. For example, motor stiffness would reduce the body's response to a frightening stimulus, and would also reduce the enactment of fear in response to thinking about (i.e. internally modelling) a frightening stimulus. This might be regarded as beneficial in states where emotions are pathologically debilitating.

However, this emotional blunting would also apply to pleasurable and gratifying stimuli, so that actually being offered a prestigious job might fail to provoke the usual gratifying feelings, and certainly the *prospect* of getting a prestigious job would fail to induce happiness. Failure to feel gratification in response to anticipated events is a plausible cause of demotivation, which is another recognised undesirable effect of neuroleptics, and it would be a consequence of being unable to anticipate events with a sense of pleasure.

Usually, thinking about (i.e. internally modelling) events leading up to personal success will lead to the enactment of a physical sensation of happiness (e.g. the glow of pleasure as we imagine receiving a Nobel Prize...). This 'here-and-now' pleasure helps to keep us working towards remote goals. By contrast, motivation is less powerful if the prospect of success does not bring with it any here-and-now reward of pleasurable sensation.

Testing this theory would depend upon distinguishing and measuring the different clinical effects of drugs – for example, discriminating between the motor effects of old-style neuroleptics, and the therapeutic effects of sedation caused by the newer 'atypical' drugs. In so far as the atypical drugs do not have motor side-effects, they are probably not really neuroleptics. Instead, their activity probably depends on their excellent hypnotic properties – as was argued in previous chapters, deep and restorative sleep can be of considerable benefit in many psychotic illnesses.

The conclusion is that neuroleptic drugs are a double-edged sword. In a nutshell, they seem to operate by immobilising muscles and thereby blunting emotion. The effect is almost always regarded as unpleasant by healthy people, because pleasant emotions are blunted along with unpleasant ones. This may explain why neuroleptic drugs are virtually never abused – they are very unpleasant to take. However, when a person is dominated by unpleasant emotions, ideas and sensations, then this emotional blunting is very welcome.

Unfortunately, the positive effect of dulling the angst of unpleasant emotions with neuroleptics can seldom be obtained without the negative effect of blunting pleasant emotions. This emphasises the fact that the dosage is absolutely critical, and should be carefully and individually adjusted to balance the benefits and drawbacks in the most favourable direction possible.

Sedatives as a treatment for mania – the 'atypical neuroleptics'

Most neuroleptics are sedatives as well as being specifically neuroleptic – in other words, they reduce arousal and make patients sleepy. Their hypnotic effect may be particularly useful in full-blown mania, as it has been argued above that delirium is an important aspect of the psycho-pathology. When chronic and severe sleep deprivation is a critical factor in pathogenesis, the induction of sleep may be curative.

Interestingly, sedatives were used to control mania before the invention of neuroleptics. Examples would include such nineteenth-century drugs as bromide and paraldehyde, and subsequently the barbiturates. However, sedatives were probably used in divided daily doses in order to make manic patients so drowsy that they could not move – a crude and undesirable method of controlling behaviour.

However, it is possible that sedation and reduction of arousal have a genuine therapeutic effect of their own. The value of non-neuroleptic sedatives is currently recognised in that a combination of low-dose neuroleptic and a benzodia-zepine (e.g. lorazepam) is currently a standard treatment for acute manic episodes. This practice implicitly acknowledges that the neuroleptic and sedative effects are potentially dissociable, and are both desirable.

If sleep deprivation is recognised as a major factor in full-blown, psychotic mania, then the induction of sustained sleep becomes a major priority. This would imply that sedative drugs should be given in a single large dose at night, rather than being spread evenly in divided doses throughout the day. As noted above, a 'good night's sleep' sometimes has an immediate effect in terminating psychotic symptoms in mania.

Another alternative is ECT, which is immediately benefi-cial in many cases of mania – producing an instant resolu-tion of or substantial improvement in psychotic symptoms such as jumbled speech, hearing voices or grandiose delusions. I have argued elsewhere in this book that ECT is an anti-delirium intervention which exerts its therapeutic effect by inducing a state equivalent to deep sleep (the important factor is probably the post-ictal sleep, rather than the epileptic fit itself).

The wheel turns? Anti-epileptic sedatives and mania

Recently, the anti-epileptic drugs carbamazepine (Tegretol) and sodium valproate (Epilim) have been used as 'mood stabilisers' to prevent manic episodes. These seem to be effective in some patients, but again their mode of action is not known. It may be that the anti-epileptics are working merely as sedatives and hypnotics – to reduce arousal, decrease anxiety and promote sleep. In other words, anti-epileptic drugs may work in a manner that differs very little from the action of benzodiazepines, or indeed the older tranquillising drugs such as barbiturates, paraldehyde or bromide – drugs which are also anti-epileptic.

Perhaps the treatment of mania is turning full circle, with an increased understanding of how to use sedatives in treatment – and the next step is prevention. As sleep deprivation has such an important role in causing mania, it could be speculated that mania may be prevented by hypnotics alone, ensuring a good night's sleep, especially when arousal levels are high and fatigue is low.

Neuroleptics and lithium can both have dangerous side-effects, and their emotionally blunting action may be demotivating in some individuals. The possibility of replacing lithium and neuroleptics by sedatives, either for the treatment of an acute manic episode, or for the prevention of recurrent episodes, would certainly constitute progress, even if (as is probable) this therapeutic option proved to be effective in only a certain proportion of patients.

Lithium – a different kind of 'neuroleptic'

One of the most mysterious drugs in modern psychiatry is lithium. It is simply a metal ion, and it is given as a simple salt such as lithium carbonate. Initially, lithium was given to manic patients as a treatment for acute mania, in which it seemed to have calming and sedating effects rather like the neuroleptics. Nowadays it is more often given (in lower doses) to *prevent* attacks of mania and depression in patients diagnosed as suffering from 'bipolar affective disorder' (more often termed 'manic-depressive' illness) who are prone to frequent and severe attacks of mania and depression.

At present it seems uncertain what lithium achieves therapeutically in either a pharmacological or a psychological sense. If taken prophylactically, lithium reduces the frequency and severity of manic attacks, but how it does this is a mystery. The usual perception is that apart from its side-effects (tremor, thirst, etc.), lithium has no effect on a person's state of mind, cognition or emotion.

However, on specific questioning most lithium users are insistent that lithium 'irons out' the usual ups and downs of mood, so that they feel both less sad and less happy. Thus lithium affects 'normal' emotions as well as the extreme emotions of mania and depression. In other words, the 'mood-stabilising' effect of lithium sounds very like a mild neuroleptic-like *blunting of emotions*.

Neuroleptics can be used to treat acute depression as well as mania, and are also often effective preventive drugs both for recurrent mania and for depression – the similarities between neuroleptics and lithium are indeed striking. Both produce similar EEG changes, and both classes act on the basal ganglia that control precise movements – although lithium produces a rapid tremor, which is distinct from the Parkinsonian side-effects of neuroleptics.

My suggestion is that we should conceptualise lithium as a mild quasi neuroleptic – that is, it is a neuroleptic in terms of its clinical action in blunting emotion, although it is not chemically a neuroleptic. Like neuroleptics, lithium probably prevents the enactment of emotional body states by affecting the basal ganglia, but unlike the neuroleptics it does this in a way that holds the musculature such that a tremor is produced rather than tonic contraction and stiffness. Lithium also has the further advantage of avoiding the long-term, probably neurotoxic, side-effect of tardive dyskinesia.

Thus lithium probably prevents mania by preventing or damping the 'high' state of arousal that initiates the manic sequence. This means that, when given chronically, lithium is not really a prophylactic, at least not in the way it is usually considered to be prophylactic. Rather, it is a continuously given acute treatment, and the clinical effect of lithium in mania is to 'calm' excited states by means akin (but not identical) to neuroleptics, as was recognised when the drug was first introduced and used to treat acute manic episodes.

When given chronically to prevent mania, lithium is actually being used in a manner closely analogous to the use of chronic low-dose neuroleptics for the prevention of schizophrenic breakdowns – for example, when neuroleptics are given as a 'depot' injection. Like neuroleptics, lithium probably has the therapeutic action of blunting emotions, and this blunting is not an accidental or unwanted 'side-effect' of the drug, but is intrinsic to its ability to reduce the frequency and severity of episodes of mania (and depression). People who are prone to large emotional swings may be grateful to have these confined within narrower boundaries, and lithium can achieve this. Whether or not lithium is taken should not be decided on the basis of whether patients have a formal diagnosis of 'bipolar affective disorder'. Rather, it should rest on whether patients have a better quality of life on the drug than without it.

If blunting of emotion is the primary therapeutic effect of lithium, then it would make sense to titrate the dose of lithium against its effects on emotion. At present, lithium dose is not titrated against clinical effect, but is kept within a safe 'window' by repeated blood sampling. This 'black-box', all-or-nothing approach to lithium dosage was inevitable, given that there was no understanding of how lithium worked. The dose of lithium was seen to represent only one of three possibilities (based on blood levels), namely too low and ineffective, too high and toxic, or acceptably within the effective and non-toxic range. However, it may be possible (and safer) to give lower doses than those usually considered to be the minimum effective dose in patients whose clinical response of mood-blunting is apparent, even when the blood level is below the usual 'effective' window.

The aim of lithium prophylaxis should be to achieve an *optimal* degree of emotional blunting that provides the maximum therapeutic benefit in terms of reducing the risk of relapse compared to the minimum demotivation at minimum risk of other undesirable effects (e.g. tremor, thirst, renal toxicity). People should feel better overall when taking lithium than they do without it, and they ought to feel that the benefits of blunting aversive emotions and preventing extreme emotions more than compensate for the cost of 'taking the top off' gratifying emotions.

Again, temperament and individual disposition are important. However, for many people lithium prophylactic therapy will inevitably be a trade-off between good and bad psychological effects, and they will not be able to have one without the other.

CHAPTER TWELVE

Schizophrenia

Schizophrenia is the term given to patients suffering psychiatric illnesses that the general public would consider to be the classic form of 'madness' – a person roaming the streets conversing with imaginary voices, shouting strange ideas, talking nonsense and adopting bizarre postures. Delusions are prominent, and often constitute 'paranoid' ideas of self-reference in which patients see themselves as being at the centre of some large scheme or conspiracy which is often hostile, making regular references to them in the newspapers and broadcast media.

The diagnosis of schizophrenia dates back 100 years to the work of Emil Kraepelin, who coined the term 'dementia praecox' and drew attention to the long-term and progressive decline in function. The term 'schizophrenia' was introduced by Eugene Bleuler to refer to the 'splitting' of affect from other psychological functions leading to a dissociation between the social situation and the emotion expressed. Nowadays, schizophrenia is a syndromal diagnosis that is made on the basis of long-term psychotic symptoms which occur in 'clear consciousness'.

People who are diagnosed as schizophrenic (in the UK) probably include some of the most severe and chronic psychiatric patients, in the sense that the diagnosis of schizophrenia is associated with a profound disintegration of personality. Schizophrenics include many individuals who experience a long-term and usually incurable illness, and whose personality and lifestyle undergo a qualitative, permanent and tragic decline. The diagnostic category of schizophrenia is, in a sense, the most important of all psychiatric diagnoses, because it represents the classic form of functional psychosis, constitutes a major element of the workload of traditional asylum psychiatrists, and stands at the very heart of the dominant nosology.

However, whether this group of patients can reasonably be regarded as constituting a single, coherent biological category is extremely doubtful.

The nature of schizophrenia

It is part of the argument of this book that acute schizophrenia is essentially indistinguishable from acute mania and agitated delirium. The three cannot be separated on the basis of examination of a patient in an acute state over a few days. Instead, the diagnosis of schizophrenia is made on the basis of the long-term events and outcome of the illness. A patient is only given the diagnosis of schizophrenia if they have been psychotic for a period of several months without recovering. By the time they have attracted the diagnosis of schizophrenia, they will have become part of a group with a generally poor prognosis. By contrast, manic patients are those with a relapsing and remitting course (with complete recovery between episodes), and the diagnosis of delirium is made when a physical cause (such as drug intoxication) exists, and there is swift and complete recovery following removal of this cause. (There is a further, slightly unrespectable diagnostic category of 'psychogenic' psychosis, which is made when a person breaks down following extreme 'stress' – and which I would suggest is usually an acute agitated delirium caused by sleep deprivation.)

Thus schizophrenia is a diagnosis that refers to a group of patients with long-term hallucinations, delusions and thought disorder. In addition, patients frequently suffer from a progressive 'dementing' process which affects personality, social behaviour and cognitive function ('dementia praecox' means 'precocious dementia'). Broadly speaking, schizophrenia emerges in young adulthood with a gradual accumulation of dementing 'negative' symptoms such as social withdrawal, lack of emotional reactivity, lack of drive and decline in intellectual ability. The idea is that schizophrenia is a disease in which there is progressive brain damage (with causes that may perhaps be genetic, infective or traumatic), and this brain damage renders the patient more susceptible to acute psychotic episodes.

I have described a caricature of a person with schizophrenia, but it is more difficult to provide any unitary account of the nature of schizophrenia. It is impossible to answer the question 'What *is* schizophrenia?' on the basis of a purely syndromal diagnosis. The symptoms and signs are neither causally related to one another, nor related to an underlying pathology. Most of the current would-be unifying theories are at the level of suggested neurotransmitter abnormalities. However, neurotransmitter changes are not diagnosable in living humans, and in any case neurotransmitter changes do not explain what is going on at the psychological level, as the intervening links of the causal chain are unspecified.

Even more fundamentally, it is not at all clear that schizophrenia is 'one thing', has one cause or represents a useful delineation. It has long been a truism in some circles that schizophrenia is a collection of separate pathological processes leading to a uniform type of illness. I was taught this 20 years ago, so the idea is hardly novel. According to this view, rather like 'heart failure', schizophrenia can be regarded as describing a pathological end-state of several diseases, rather than a disease in itself. Certainly 'schizophrenic' patients differ widely in their clinical features, in their response to treatment, and in their long-term natural history. Unfortunately, so do the end-state pathological findings. For instance, there is no characteristic brain abnormality from which schizophrenia could be diagnosed. Contrary to what was hoped 20 years ago, schizophrenia does not appear to be characterised by any specific pathological end-state. Brain abnormalities are non-specific and do not clearly discriminate schizophrenic patients from those with other psychiatric illnesses or from normal control subjects.

Despite widespread tacit acknowledgment of the heterogeneity of the diagnostic category, most schizophrenia research (and clinical practice) continues to talk of the syndrome as if it were a unitary disease that might have a single cause, a single pathology and a single treatment. There has been little attempt to subdivide schizophrenia into its proper biological and psychological categories.

The most fruitful strategy for approaching schizophrenia would be to discover the *pathological processes* which are at work in the type of patients who currently attract a diagnosis of schizophrenia, and to link these to the psychological abnormalities that are observed. This turns out to be much easier than might be anticipated. When this happens, schizophrenia becomes a different proposition, and quite novel strategies for treatment become plausible.

Schizophrenic delusions – theory-of-mind delusions

First, let us consider schizophrenic delusions. It has already been argued that delusions fall into at least two classes. There is a class of false, unshakable, dominating beliefs about the dispositions, motivations and intentions of others that form the category which I have termed 'theory-of-mind' delusions – for example, persecutory, jealous and erotomaniac delusions. Such delusions can be found in people with no cognitive abnormalities, in whom these 'pure cases' are termed delusional disorder.

Some schizophrenic delusional beliefs fit this 'theory-of-mind' category – for example, long-term delusions of persecution based on the belief that a person or group is hostile. As they are not associated with pathological cognition, we would expect such beliefs to be resistant to persuasion, resistant to drug treatment, and to be present even during remissions of the long-term psychotic illness. Probably these theory-of-mind delusions are a consequence of the affective abnormalities found in some patients who are diagnosed as schizophrenic.

For example, I have seen persecutory delusions develop before my eyes as a patient became more and more fearful following a reduction in the dose of neuroleptic medication.

This patient had a pre-existing belief in the ill will of social workers. This belief was present at all times, but when he was well the belief was neither dominant nor distressing. However, after reduction of the neuroleptic dose, the patient's level of fear gradually escalated (as the emotionally blunting effects began to wear off). At first the patient became perplexed – fearful and suspicious, but uncertain of the reason for this. Increasing perplexity was apparently a result of trying to understand what was going on, perhaps exacerbated by a mild degree of cognitive impairment which made it difficult to think things through.

At a certain point, this patient crossed a line and became convinced that the cause of his growing fear was increasing persecution by the team social workers – people whose motives he had long suspected. Suddenly everything made sense, and the belief that the social workers were persecuting him came to dominate his waking life, and was used to explain all manner of problems and frustrations. When a social worker called round to his flat, or was spotted nearby, this was taken as evidence that they were spying and collecting data. In a sense, of course, all of this was true, and the social workers were indeed observing, collecting and pooling data. However, what was misunderstood was the *motivation* of the social workers, as the patient thought that they were engaged in establishing enough evidence to lock him up permanently (an interpretation which was, of course, untrue).

When the dose of neuroleptic was increased, the patient's arousal and fear diminished, intense but unpleasant emotions were blunted, and the intensity of the belief in persecution also waned until it ceased to dominate. Eventually the patient was left with his long-standing suspicion of social workers, but with no overtly false beliefs.

The lesson that this example is intended to reinforce is that the false beliefs that characterise theory-of-mind delusions are not wholly treatable by medication, and indeed the false beliefs themselves should not be the focus of treatment. It would have been a serious mistake to keep raising the dose of neuroleptic in an attempt to eradicate all suspicions and false beliefs about social workers, since these were not based on pathological cognition. Rather, what was treatable and also served as the focus of treatment was to ameliorate the fearful emotional state that both drove and was a consequence of the false beliefs.

Once established, a theory-of-mind delusion cannot usually be eradicated, although medication may be effective in diminishing the emotional drive to act upon that belief. However, this occurs at a cost. The emotion-blunting action of neuroleptics means that this class of drugs has the potential to operate in a generally demotivating fashion. When a patient is dominated by unpleasant emotions, this can benefit their overall clinical state. In normal controls, demotivation is unpleasant and may be debilitating. Thus a patient's overall clinical state, their happiness and social adjustment, are the appropriate outcome measures against which drug dosage should be titrated – *not* the presence of a specific false belief.

Schizophrenic delusions – bizarre delusions

However, as well as theory-of-mind delusions, based on mistaken inferences concerning other people's intentions, motivations and dispositions, and fuelled by affective changes, schizophrenic patients more characteristically also suffer what have been termed 'bizarre' delusions. Bizarre delusions can be defined as delusions which are based upon illogical, incoherent or incomprehensible reasoning processes. Because the chain of inference leading up to them is illogical, the beliefs which emerge as a consequence of this type of reasoning are often impossible propositions – bizarre delusions.

For example, I once spoke with a patient who believed that she was under surveillance by some kind of laser beams, and that these were used to project up large television pictures of her. She told me that, as we were speaking together, her neighbours several miles away were also sitting around watching a gigantic television picture of the two of us speaking. Other patients have complained that their minds were being read, or that their thoughts were being somehow extracted, or alien thoughts inserted – again by some vaguely defined technology such as radar or lasers.

Such beliefs are usually a consequence of a sequence of inference which is similar to dream logic, and the beliefs are never properly worked out or argued. As mentioned previously, the reason for this is that bizarre delusions are a consequence of delirium – they proceed by dream logic because they are almost literally dreams. Bizarre delusions are remembered dreams that break through into consciousness as a consequence of fluctuating levels of consciousness.

It is suggested that patients suffering from bizarre delusions are in an abnormal state of consciousness, fluctuating between delirium and waking, and therefore functionally brain-impaired. This ought to be apparent from serial EEGs as well as from observing the clinical signs and symptoms of delirium.

Because bizarre delusions are a consequence of delirium, they are potentially completely curable if the delirium can be treated. If a remission is achieved, then the patients should completely lose their bizarre delusions, unlike their theory-of-mind delusions.

Schizophrenic hallucinations

Hearing voices is one of the classic symptoms of madness. Specifically, hallucinations *in clear consciousness* are said to be a sign of psychotic illnesses such as schizophrenia, mania and severe depression. However, the definition of 'clear' consciousness is contestable in schizophrenia, and I have suggested that acute schizophrenia is a delirious state.

The pathological mechanism by which hallucinations might arise in clear consciousness has never been satisfactorily elucidated. Various ingenious hypotheses have been devised to explain why it is that schizophrenic patients are unable to distinguish the 'inner voices' of auditory hallucinations from the external voices of other people. However, none of these hypotheses seem convincing from a biological perspective.

I suggest that hallucinations do *not* occur in clear consciousness, but that they only occur in a delirious state of impaired consciousness. I also suggest that 'schizophrenic' patients with bizarre delusions will be found to have impaired consciousness. It is the diagnosis of clear consciousness that is at fault in schizophrenia.

After all, hallucinations are not unusual – many normal people have experienced them, but only in states of impaired consciousness. This is particularly true of hypnagogic or hypnopompic hallucinations which occur when people are drowsily falling asleep or waking up. These hallucinations can be auditory (e.g. voices speaking short phrases, shouting, thumps and other noises) or visual (e.g. shapes or movements). Such hallucinations therefore happen when people have 'clouded consciousness' and are not quite awake or alert. They are probably fragments of dreams that break through into normal waking awareness as consciousness fluctuates.

Other people have experienced auditory or visual hallucinations when delirious with a high fever, sunstroke, or something similar. In addition, many people deliberately induce visions, voices and hallucinations in other sensory modalities by taking drugs such as LSD. There are many types of hallucinatory state which depend on the drug being taken, but the common feature of all these hallucinations is functional brain impairment (i.e. delirium).

It seems overwhelmingly likely that hallucinations (e.g. auditory, visual or somatic hallucinations) that occur in patients diagnosed as suffering from 'schizophrenia' are also the consequence of delirium. In other words, hallucinations in schizophrenics are *not* occurring 'in clear consciousness'. The idea that hallucinations can occur in clear consciousness is again an artefact of too insensitive a diagnosis of delirium, which fails to use the most accurate test (serial EEGs).

Hallucinations also lead to bizarre delusions as people try to explain their imagined physical experiences. For example, delusions such as that in which a person's thoughts are being 'withdrawn' from their head, or in which alien thoughts are inserted, or in which their body is being controlled, are possible consequences of physical hallucinations of the sense of touch. Similarly, the senses of smell and taste can be subject to hallucinations.

Acute schizophrenia is a delirious state

If a more valid clinical diagnosis of delirium was to be adopted, it would be predicted that any schizophrenic patient who exhibits bizarre delusions, hallucinations or the kind of jumbled or nonsensical speech which is considered to characterise 'thought disorder' would be diagnosed as delirious.

The cause of the delirium in such a patient might be any insult to the brain (i.e. infective, inflammatory, toxic or – like psychosis in mania or depression – sleep deprivation). Thus any likely cause of delirium should be searched for and treated if possible – with chronic, severe sleep deprivation being a likely candidate in many instances. Induction of sleep with either drugs or ECT may provide rapid benefit.

However, patients who attract a diagnosis of schizophrenia are, by definition, those in a poor-prognosis group. Moreover, it is known that the effect of any potential cause of delirium is exacerbated when acting upon an abnormal brain. For example, delirium is commonest in patients at the extremes of the lifespan – with either immature or senile brains – and in patients with Alzheimer's dementia or multi-infarct dementia. It is highly likely that a proportion of patients with schizophrenia have abnormal brains of various types, probably due to a variety of progressive dementing processes that have not yet been identified and classified. More needs to be said about this.

Negative symptoms

Negative symptoms are so called because they are *reductions* in normal behaviour, or absences of behaviour – while hallucinations, thought disorder and delusions are considered to be positive symptoms in the sense that they *add* to normal behaviour. The negative symptoms of schizophrenia include lack of emotion and 'flat' mood ('affective blunting'), lack of motivation ('avolia'), 'asocial' behaviour in which the patient avoids other people, and 'alogia' or poverty of thought (which means that the person speaks very little, and so far as anyone can tell also *thinks* very little).

The negative symptoms of schizophrenia are cognitive and behavioural abnormalities that are probably the consequence of a progressive brain abnormality or dementia – dementia being a *generalised* intellectual and behavioural decline, usually due to structural brain abnormalities. However, there is a potentially very worrying overlap between deterioration due to presumed dementing processes, and an almost identical deterioration due to the neuroleptic drugs that are used to treat patients who are prone to acute psychotic breakdowns.

The picture of a patient with prominent negative symptoms is of a strangely behaving person (usually a man) who leads an isolated life, talking to few people and showing little desire to talk, perhaps nocturnally awake and wandering and sleeping by day, but doing very little and without any ambition. There will usually be hallucinations such that the patient can be seen to react to voices by muttering or shouting back at them. There may be a strange way of walking or strange postures adopted. Acute episodes with agitated behaviour and exacerbations of hallucinations and delusions may occur from time to time. Little information can be obtained at interview, but there may be evidence of delusions, strange beliefs, and reports of strange perceptions of influenced thinking and body sensations. A considerable range of structural brain abnormalities (usually quantitatively rather than qualitatively abnormal) may be seen either on a brain scan or when the brain is examined after death.

Such a picture may progressively worsen over time and be essentially permanent and irreversible – at any rate, negative symptoms do not respond to the same treatment as positive symptoms. Indeed, negative symptoms (e.g. demotivation and emotional blunting) are usually made worse by neuroleptics, and it is possible that in some patients negative symptoms may be substantially *caused by* neuroleptics. As discussed previously, neuroleptics probably blunt emotions by an action on the basal ganglia. This blunting is beneficial in the case of pathological aversive emotions such as fear, but unfortunately neuroleptics also blunt pleasurable emotions. Moreover, it is plausible that a blunting of pleasurable emotions *could* cause all of the negative symptoms of schizophrenia.

A patient who is unable to experience normal pleasure from social interactions will tend to avoid them. In particular, when pleasurable emotions cannot be enacted in response to anticipation, then motivation may be severely damaged – thoughts of the future do not lead to gratifying feelings in the here and now, so it is difficult to make oneself embark on any long-term projects. Without the inbuilt system for generating rewarding emotions, thinking becomes an activity that lacks reward, reality seems abstract and distant, and a negative, inert and placid life dedicated to avoiding unpleasant emotions offers the greatest satisfaction. This situation may be exacerbated if patients on neuroleptics are also suffering the extremely unpleasant side-effect of akathesia, a state of psychological and physical restlessness which may itself tend to provoke a reaction of social withdrawal.

Therefore it seems likely that patients diagnosed as schizophrenic and suffering from 'negative symptoms' represent at least two groups, namely those who are suffering from some kind of dementia which may be progressive and permanent, and those whose negative symptoms are a side-effect of neuroleptics. The important thing is not to misdiagnose patients whose negative symptoms are drug-induced, as these symptoms are potentially reversible.

Patients vary widely in their sensitivity to neuroleptic drugs, there is considerable variation with regard to which drugs suit which people, and different doses are required for acute and long-term use. Individual tailoring of treatment and dose will almost certainly be necessary. The aim of long-term treatment should be to suppress positive symptoms with the minimum of negative symptoms. When the dose is correct, the patient should feel better overall –

that is, the benefits of treatment should outweigh the disadvantages.

Thus negative symptoms can often be treated. A minimum dose can be sought, or one of the 'atypical' neuroleptics can be tried – these are probably only very weakly neuroleptic at the recommended doses, but act mainly as hypnotics. It seems very likely that the schizophrenic patients whose negative symptoms were apparently cured by clozapine were in fact benefiting from withdrawal of neuroleptics and loss of their drug-induced negative symptoms. Even among chronic schizophrenics who have not had a remission for decades, remarkable recoveries *sometimes* occur.

Schizophrenia is not a unified biological entity

The clinical picture of schizophrenia is therefore a variable mixture of delirium superimposed on dementia with the possible complication of neuroleptic side-effects. There is really no good scientific reason to assume that the many and varied symptoms of schizophrenia can be attributed to a single cause.

Nor is the diagnosis of schizophrenia a good guide to prognosis, except in the crude sense that if a person has suffered symptoms without recovery for several months, then it is probable (although not certain) that they will continue to suffer similar symptoms in the long term and will not make a full recovery. Similarly, patients with a gradual (insidious) onset of symptoms without an obvious cause have a poorer prognosis than patients with an acute onset caused by some obvious and unusual 'stress'.

The diagnosis of schizophrenia is not a good guide to treatment. Some psychiatrists, encouraged by neurotransmitter theories, regard schizophrenia as a specific cerebral pathology (such as some kind of dopamine over-activity), and neuroleptics as having a specific beneficial effect on this perturbed system. However, the dopamine hypothesis of schizophrenia has never been strong, and has become progressively weaker over the years. At present the dopamine hypothesis of schizophrenia serves only to reinforce a false unitary concept of schizophrenia, and a categorical mode of treatment with neuroleptics (even in circumstances where drugs are only dubiously neuroleptic and are probably having quite different therapeutic actions).

It has often been shown that schizophrenia is best treated symptomatically. In other words, the best approach to an illness as heterogeneous as schizophrenia is probably to treat the *symptoms* that are causing the patient most concern or that are causing the greatest behavioural disruption. The diagnosis tells you less than the symptoms about the best focus for therapeutic intervention. Thus moderate agitation and preoccupation with distressing delusions or hallucinations might be treated by neuroleptics, acute agitation and dominating delusions or hallucinations might be treated by ECT, depression might be treated by antidepressants, sleeplessness by hypnotics, anxiety and fear by anxiolytics, and so on.

This symptom-focused treatment strategy is not really controversial, although it is seldom so explicit, and it strongly implies that schizophrenia is a collection of more or less coincident pathologies and symptoms. To me this suggests that 'schizophrenia' is a term which is not doing any useful work. Indeed, it is probably doing more harm than good.

A new psychiatric nosology is needed

Time to discard the diagnostic category of schizophrenia

Schizophrenia occupies a central place in the current nosology – a place which it has occupied for the past 100 years since the syndrome was delineated by Kraepelin. Yet schizophrenia is neither biologically valid nor clinically useful as a diagnostic category. When classification is mistaken, then research based upon it is bound to be wrong because the information has been collected for groups of dissimilar patients. Reform of nosology is therefore a prerequisite for valid psychiatric research.

Schizophrenia is a very old diagnosis, and most 100-year-old diagnoses in other more highly developed branches of medicine were long ago superseded. We no longer talk about an 'ague' or a 'fever' – we talk about the infective agent, the nature of the pathological process, the specific organ affected, and the processes upon which therapeutic interventions are intended to operate. If this kind of information is not known, then people are looking for it. It is at least implicitly recognised that where there is no existing satisfactory nosology, then clinical research should be focused on devising a proper diagnostic classification.

Schizophrenia illustrates perhaps more powerfully than any other example the way in which psychiatric research and clinical progress are being thwarted by the non-biological nature of some of the diagnostic categories. So long as the categories of disease are wrong, and so long as these categories dominate research, psychiatry will be stuck at more or less its present level. Considering the vast input of research funding over a period of several decades, the clinical progress in schizophrenia has been very modest indeed, amounting to little more than a gradual process of learning how *not* to poison patients with neuroleptics. At any rate, there seems to be little doubt that the term 'schizophrenia' is now hampering effective clinical evaluation and treatment.

Factors blocking change

Unfortunately, researchers are locked into the present system by a vast infrastructure of journals, conferences and books that are wholly or partially devoted to schizophrenia research, societies of sufferers and professionals that are organised around the diagnosis, drugs marketed specifically for schizophrenia, and funding earmarked for research in this area. To reject the validity of the diagnosis of schizophrenia is to reject these sources of position, status and money. Schizophrenia is at the very heart of psychiatry both as a profession and as a research enterprise because it is *the* classic form of madness. If psychiatrists turn out to have been wrong about schizophrenia, then what else might they have been wrong about?

Psychiatrists are also sensitive to the legacy of 1960s counter-culture claims that mental illness is not real, but that it is an arbitrary method of social control. Such views are still actively propagated in the social sciences, and are influential in some of the paramedical healthcare professions. To admit that schizophrenia is a neither valid nor useful diagnostic category would be to expose the psychiatric profession to accusations of carelessness, abuse, dishonesty, incompetence and who knows what else. The position of psychiatry has never been so secure that this was felt to be a justifiable risk. Despite the existence of many eminent schizophrenia researchers who are willing, privately and off the record, to admit that the concept of schizophrenia is neither real nor useful, hardly anyone has 'broken ranks'. Official and public discourse is solidly unified in its usage of the term 'schizophrenia'.

Perhaps the hope is that schizophrenia can be discarded by stealth without anyone really noticing. Unfortunately, there seem to be no signs of this. Instead, the diagnosis carries an ever greater freight of expectation in terms of research and therapy. Articles on 'progress' in schizophrenia are regularly published in the most prestigious journals – scientific, clinical and those targeted at a lay audience. The nonsense seems invincible and immortal, and the boundary between 'normal' and 'schizophrenic' is ever more carefully patrolled, reinforcing the impression that on the one hand there are schizophrenics, and on the other there are us 'normal folk'. The two categories neither mesh nor merge.

This has to stop, and the sooner the better. The risks must be taken. Such is its rigidity of inertial misconception that progress in psychiatry depends on the complete demolition of the diagnosis of schizophrenia, and its extirpation from clinical and research discourse. From the rubble of schizophrenia we may construct a new nosology to replace the obsolete conceptions of Kraepelin.

Schizophrenia and the human condition

What is the relevance of schizophrenia to the human condition? On the face of it, schizophrenia represents something alien to the experience of normal life. What indeed is the relevance of delusional disorder, depression and mania? And why have I re-explained these disorders using concepts derived from evolutionary psychology and cognitive neuroscience?

The reason is to pave the way for a new system of classification of psychiatric illness, a new nosology based upon biologically valid psychological variables applied both to diseases and to drug effects. And the reason for this is quite simple – it is to free psychiatry from its current conceptual stasis and force the subject to emerge from the intellectual ghetto it has occupied for several decades.

While it has been occupying this Kraepelinian prison, psychiatry has learned virtually nothing from biology, and has made no substantial contribution to the rest of science at all. It is a pitiful record of misplaced activity, the failure of which has been blurred but not obscured by vast efforts at public relations and hype. We should have no regrets about leaving all of this behind, breaking down the barriers, and refreshing the subject of psychiatry by contact with the scientific disciplines outside the ghetto. There is a great deal of lost ground to make up.

The advantages of a thoroughly biological approach to psychiatric classification are that it might be expected to yield three major classes of benefit.

Research

First, it would enable research to proceed on the basis of potentially valid biological categories. This would not guarantee progress, but it would at least remove the major obstacle to progress that the present nosology represents.

Treatment

Secondly, a psychological description would in principle allow symptomatic treatment that is tailored to the individual requirements of each patient. At present each patient is categorised and their treatment determined by a psychiatric 'ghetto' diagnosis, entirely detached from any roots in the knowledge base of contemporary biological science. Instead, I propose that biologically valid psychological variables derived from evolutionary theory, neuroscience and other disciplines need to be employed. I have suggested categories such as theory-of-mind delusions as distinct from bizarre delusions, delirium measured on the basis of degrees of impaired brain function, sickness behaviour as measured on the basis of major depressive disorder, hypomania as a combination of increased arousal and analgesia, schizophrenia as various combinations of delirium and dementia, and so on.

Such a scheme allows a symptomatic *profile* of each individual patient to be built up on the basis of the presence and relative severity of these variables. A symptom-focused treatment can be tailored on an individual basis, based on knowledge of the effects of individual drugs on these symptoms – the drug effect can be individually titrated against target symptoms.

Links to normal behaviour

Thirdly, a new nosology based on psychological categories demonstrates the links between psychiatry and everyday life. To this extent, it demystifies and destigmatises psychiatric illness. Psychiatric symptoms are seen as universal aspects of the human condition, varying in their distribution and severity, but which everyone has experienced and from which no one is immune.

The world of formal psychiatric disorder and the everyday world of 'the human condition' are not separate categories, but one in which individuals occupy a moving trajectory on a constellation of biological and psychological variables. There are few aspects of formal psychiatric disorders that are completely alien to normal experience (when they are considered one at a time in their proper categories), although the combined and sustained effect is often very strange, very disturbing and very tragic.

Similarly, psychiatric drugs are regarded as members of a much broader category of agents that affect psychology, a category which includes painkillers, mild stimulants such as coffee and tea, and relaxants such as alcohol – indeed, drugs which are taken with the purpose of making life pleasanter, or at least more bearable. The drugs used to treat major psychiatric illnesses such as depression, mania and schizophrenia should, in principle, be no different. Psychotropic drugs should make patients' lives pleasanter or at least more bearable, and if they are not doing this, then hard questions must be asked about the role of psychiatric treatment and who is supposed to benefit from it.

In this sense, formal psychiatric disorder has much to teach us about how to cope with the human condition – how to make the best of our lives.

And it is to this topic of how to make the best of our lives that I shall turn in the final chapter of this book.

CHAPTER THIRTEEN

Psychopharmacology and the human condition

A world of artificial gratification is upon us. The human condition is increasingly characterised by the prevalence of technological benefits, of which psychotropic drugs are only one instance. And this should be welcomed, despite the very real hazards, in the sense that the quality of life without these benefits would be diminished for nearly everyone. And for those people to whom technology provides not just alternatives, but surrogates, life might be barely worth living.

What, then, is the role of psychopharmacology in such a world – a world which we increasingly inhabit? What can psychopharmacology do to improve the human condition?

Psychopharmacological agents can help to cure illness, relieve symptoms and enhance function, allowing people to get on with their lives. It is difficult to lead a rich social life and adopt a positive view of the future when one is plagued by symptoms of malaise, exhaustion, aches and pains, or eroded by anxiety. In so far as psychopharmacology can remove these obstacles, then it should count as a boon to humankind – and one of the greatest.

For instance, analgesia is probably the most under-recognised benefit of psychopharmacology. The diminution of pain has immediate beneficial effects but, more importantly, it also enables people to achieve greater fulfilment in life. The availability of effective analgesia has significantly increased the number of days on which people such as myself (a migraine sufferer) can lead a normal life rather than lying in bed in pain.

Many people use drugs to fit themselves to the unavoidable rhythms and demands of industrial society. Without pharmacological assistance, many people would probably have to settle for lower-paid jobs, or perhaps would not be able to work at all. Drugs may provide energy or alertness on demand – for example, by the use of stimulants such as caffeine. This may be necessary when we have to cope with long hours of work, when we feel ill or tired, and when high levels of efficiency are expected. Similar benefits may be obtained from the occasional use of sleeping tablets by people whose lives disrupt their normal sleep rhythms. These are not ideal solutions to the problems of contemporary living, but they may be the best that is available.

At the other end of the emotional scale, people use recreational drugs such as alcohol to unwind and for aiding social intercourse. This anxiolytic effect is quite distinct from seeking obliterative intoxication. The contrast can be seen in southern Mediterranean countries such as Spain, where alcohol is used to lubricate personal interactions (even being taken at breakfast), yet people very seldom consume enough alcohol to become drunk. Indeed, anxiolysis is probably the most sought-after psychotropic drug effect, and alcohol the most popular of the powerful psychopharmacological agents.

So in discussing the role of psychopharmacology in relation to the human condition, the most significant point is not those drugs that make you 'high' or intoxicated, for these are more or less a sideshow – sometimes diverting and at other times destructive. The real importance lies with those drugs that have the potential to remove obstacles to fulfilment, and to give life more meaning. When they work, these agent are true 'happy pills' in the sense that they are pills which clear the path to human satisfaction.

What about the disadvantages of psychopharmacology? Effective drugs always have side-effects, there is the financial expense involved, and there is the possibility of addiction. Yet in a world where we have lost hope of political answers, there could be few things more important than technological agents which offer at least some people the possibility of a genuine enhancement of the human condition.

And the most important question about psychotropic agents should surely be that of control and access. Regulation, safety and costs naturally require consideration, but we should not lose sight of the principle that individual people who wish to avail themselves of psychopharmacological agents should have access to those agents.

The question is not whether to use psychopharmacology in pursuit of the good life – but how.

Evolution and the cognitive neuroscience of awareness, consciousness and language

What follows is the most conceptually difficult section of this book, and readers without some scientific background may have to skip it, perhaps returning to grapple with it later. They should not feel guilty about this. However, this section contains the fundamental theory of organisation of the human mind which underpins much of the argument in this book. It describes what is distinctive about human intelligence, including the evolutionary basis, nature, function and neurological mechanisms of human consciousness and language.

Consciousness is sometimes regarded as intrinsically mysterious – something probably beyond human comprehension, and perhaps even impossible to define. On the other hand, consciousness is an ordinary fact of life – babies are born without it and develop it over the first few years of life. We experience the dawn of consciousness every morning when we awaken. And whatever it is, it presumably evolved like other complex biological phenomena. Even if we regard consciousness as a curse, that in itself makes it even more plausible that it has a biological benefit to counterbalance its obvious disadvantages, otherwise natural selection would have eliminated consciousness long ago (saving a lot of hungry brain tissue in the process).

Thus consciousness cannot be any more biologically mysterious than any of the other advanced abilities – also extremely difficult to understand and explain – that we and many other animals enjoy. Indeed, consciousness is almost certainly a great deal simpler than human vision – which required enormous amounts of brain tissue and hundreds of millions of years of evolution to be perfected. Consciousness seems to have taken only tens of millions of years to develop, and involves only a relatively small amount of the cerebral cortex.

Evolution of 'awareness'

People often find 'consciousness' mysterious, but the real mystery is awareness – and many other animals are aware, so this is not a specifically human mystery.

The question of consciousness can therefore be approached by considering the general phenomenon of awareness, of which consciousness is one particular example. The mystery usually consists of puzzlement as to why humans are apparently 'conscious' (i.e. aware) of at least some of their own 'thinking' (i.e. cognitive processing), rather than cognitive processing simply generating behaviour without awareness. Why do we know that we know, instead of just knowing it? Since most of mental life (including some of the most computationally difficult tasks, such as those concerned with vision) proceeds perfectly well without awareness of processing, the question arises as to why awareness should exist at all.

Function of awareness

However, that question is badly framed. The proper question should be as follows. First, is awareness an evolved adaptation? In other words, did awareness evolve to solve a problem with reproductive consequences for the animal, or is awareness perhaps an epiphenomenon? And if we assume that awareness is an adaptation with a biologically useful function, the second question concerns the biological nature of this adaptation. What is the mechanism by which awareness solves the problem it evolved to solve?

Therefore the first difficulty with the 'mystery' of consciousness is that the question as commonly stated bundles together several questions that need to be considered separately. There is the general phenomenon of awareness, and consciousness is 'merely' a specific type of awareness. In fact, consciousness is awareness of inner body states, as will be described later.

Awareness is not unique to humans – many animals display the characteristics of awareness, and it is something that seems to have evolved many times in many lineages. Moreover, awareness has a quite precise definition – it is the ability to direct attention selectively to specific aspects of the environment, and to be able to manipulate these aspects cognitively over a more prolonged time scale than normal cognitive processing will allow (i.e. to hold in mind selected aspects of the perceptual landscape).

Technically, awareness is attention plus working memory (i.e. the ability to attend selectively to a range of perceived stimuli and a short-term memory store into which several of these attended items can be 'loaded', held simultaneously, and combined). Awareness is a standard variable in psychological research, and can be unproblematically measured in, for example, animal vision. It is studied by methods such as measurement of performance on memory tasks while monitoring gaze direction, delaying responses and recording brain activity. When brain activity correlates exactly with performance of tasks, then it can be assumed that that part of the brain is involved in that particular task. Moreover, the length of time for which brain activity is sustained corresponds to an animal's ability to 'hold in mind' information for immediate use. Researchers are therefore recording the operation of a temporary store.

Awareness is thus not an aspect of *social* intelligence. Instead, awareness is a mechanism of integration. It is a way of converging and combining information, and it is a functional ability that is found in complex animals living in complex environments. Awareness therefore relates to the ability to cope with complexity of perception and behaviour, and it is found not only in social animals, but also in solitary animals. Although awareness is found in animals right across the animal kingdom, *consciousness* has a much more limited distribution. I suggest that consciousness is probably confined to a small number of recently evolved social animals such as the great ape lineage (especially common chimpanzees and bonobos) and perhaps a few other recently evolved social mammals (e.g. elephants and dolphins).

Awareness is located in working memory

Awareness consists of attention and working memory (WM). For someone to be aware of a perception, it must be selectively attended to, and the representation of that entity must be kept active and held in the brain for a sufficient length of time to allow other cognitive representations to interact with it, and in a place where other cognitive representations can be projected. Working memory is such a place, where information converges and is kept active for longer periods than usual. Hence *working memory* is the anatomical site of awareness.

The nature of working memory can be understood using concepts derived from cognitive neuroscience. Working memory is a three-dimensional space filled with neurones that can activate in patterns. Cognition is conceptualised as the processing of information in the form of topographically organised (three-dimensional) patterns of neural activity called *representations*, because each specific pattern 'represents' a perceptual input. Thus seeing a particular shape produces a pattern of cell activation on the retina, and this shape is reproduced, summarised, transformed, combined, etc., in patterns of cell activation in the visual system of the brain. Each pattern of brain-cell activation in each visual region then retains a formal relationship to the original retinal activation.

Representations are the units of thinking. In the visual system there may be representations of the colour, movement and shading of an object, each of these having been constructed from information extracted from the original pattern of cell activation in the retina (using many built-in and learned assumptions about the nature of the visual world). The propagation and combination of representations is the process of cognition.

Cognitive representations in most parts of the brain typically stay active and persist for a time scale of the order of several *tens* of milliseconds. However, in WM cognitive representations may be maintained over a much longer time scale – perhaps *hundreds* or *thousands* of milliseconds – and probably by the action of specialised 'delay' neurones which maintain firing over longer periods. So WM is a three-dimensional space which contains patterns of nerve firing that are sustained long enough for them to interact with other 'incoming' patterns. This sustaining of cognitive representations means that WM is also a 'convergence' region which brings together and integrates highly processed data from several separate information streams.

Any animal that is able selectively to attend to and sustain cognitive representations could be said to possess a WM and to be 'aware' – although the content of that awareness and the length of time for which it can be sustained may be simple and short, respectively. The capacity of WM will certainly vary between species, and the structures that perform the function of WM will vary substantially according to the design of the central nervous system. In other words, WM is a function which is performed by structures that have arisen by convergent evolution. It is not homologous between all animals that possess it – presumably the large and effective WM of an octopus is performed by quite different brain structures to WM in a sheep-dog, structures that have no common ancestor and evolved down quite different paths. The mechanism and connectivity of the *human* WM allows cognitive representations from different perceptual modalities or from different attended parts of the environment to be kept active simultaneously, to interact, and to undergo integration in order to enable the production of appropriate whole-organism behavioural responses.

Working memory is reciprocally linked to long-term memory (LTM), such that representations formed in WM can be stored in LTM as patterns of enhanced or impaired transmission between nerve cells (the mechanism by which this occurs is uncertain, but probably involves a structure called the hippocampus). Thus temporary patterns of active nerves are converted to much more lasting patterns of easier or more difficult transmission *between* nerves. The patterns in LTM may be later recalled and re-evoked in WM for further cycles of processing and elaboration.

This is how complex thinking gets done – a certain maximum number of representations can interact in WM in the time available (perhaps several seconds). Therefore there is a limit to what can be done in WM during the span of activation of its representations. To do more requires storing the intermediate steps in reasoning. The products of an interaction in WM can be summarised ('chunked') and 'posted' to LTM, where they wait until they are needed again. When they have been recalled and reactivated, these complex packaged representations from LTM can undergo further cycles of interaction and modification, each building up the complexity of representations and conceptual thought.

WM is therefore conceptualised as a site for the integration of attended perceptual information deriving from a range of sensory inputs. Awareness seems to be used to select and integrate relevant inputs from a complex environment to enable animals to choose from a large repertoire of behavioural responses. There is a selective pressure to evolve WM in any animal that is capable of complex behavioural responses to a complexly variable environment. Thus the cognitive representations in WM in non-conscious animals are derived from *external* sensory inputs (e.g. vision, hearing, smell, taste and touch).

The critical point for this current argument is that non-conscious animals may be aware of their surroundings, but they lack the capacity to be aware of their own *body states*. Awareness of the outer environment is common, but awareness of inner body states is unique to conscious animals.

Evolution of 'consciousness'

Awareness of body states

The starting point for evolution of consciousness is thus an aware animal with an integration centre called working memory which is able to maintain the activity of attended perceptual representations. The evolutionary breakthrough to consciousness occurs when WM receives not just external perceptual information from the senses, but also projections of inner body states. In other words, in a conscious animal WM contains body-state representations as well as perceptions of the external environment.

Consciousness arises when body-state information becomes accessible to awareness. And consciousness depends on the animal evolving the ability to feed information on its internal physiological state into WM, so that it can be integrated with sensory perceptual information.

First, some terminology needs to be introduced. The physiological state of the body constitutes what is more commonly called an *emotion*. To put it another way, emotions are body states as they are represented in the brain. Damasio has pointed out that although we think of the brain as being concerned mainly with processing information derived from inputs by the five senses, in fact the control of *internal* body states is the primary evolutionary function of the brain. The primitive brain in lower animals is mainly a device for monitoring what is going on in the body – brains (or rather a central nervous system) evolved when bodies got too large to allow communication to occur purely by diffusion of chemicals. Therefore the main business of the brain is to monitor and interpret body states (including emotions), and to modulate these states.

Feelings is the term used to refer to emotions of which we are aware. For instance, 'fear' is activation of the sympathetic nervous system and preparation of the body for 'fight or flight' – so fear refers to the effects of the sympathetic nervous system on the disposition of internal organs ('viscera') such as muscle tension, heart rate, sweat glands, and so on. When these body states register in the brain and affect behaviour *without* awareness, this can be termed the *emotion* of fear. When we become aware that we are frightened, this is termed the *feeling* of fear.

By this account, emotions may be non-conscious, while feelings are conscious. Emotions are found in many animals, most of which are not conscious and are unaware of their emotions. A cow can experience the emotion of fear (and react appropriately) but it will not have the feeling of fear – it will not know that it is frightened, it will just *be* frightened. In other words, fear does not have a representation in the WM of a cow. By contrast, a person can experience fear either without or with awareness. Fear is present when the body state of fear is present, but humans may or may not have awareness of this – a person can be frightened without knowing it, just as a cow can. For example, when watching a horror film and absorbed in the action, a person might experience the physiological state of fear (e.g. thumping heart, hair standing on end – a preparation for action). However, they may lack awareness of the fact that they are frightened until such time as they are interrupted and asked whether they are frightened – at which point an awareness of fear is produced (an awareness of tense posture, creeping skin, hair standing on end, etc.).

Thus fear can be an emotion, leading to an adaptive behaviour such as fight or flight – and the behaviour may occur without a person having any awareness of their inner state. However, in conscious animals such as humans there may also be awareness of an inner state – the person may know that they are scared. The question is, what is the use of knowing that one is frightened? What is the adaptive function of consciousness – especially given that most animals function perfectly well without such knowledge? What function did consciousness evolve to perform?

The answer is that consciousness is an aspect of social intelligence, and the adaptive function of consciousness is to enable the cognitive modelling of social situations. Animals evolved the ability to project body-state representations into working memory so that emotions could interact with perceptions. Awareness of inner body states is an accidental by-product of bringing together cognitive representations of emotions and cognitive representations of *social* perceptions in working memory.

Working memory as a convergence zone for emotions and perceptions

Consciousness therefore exists because WM is the location – and the *only* location – where the streams of internal and external information converge, where information about the environment is juxtaposed with information about the body, and where emotional representations can interact with, modify and *evaluate* representations of social perceptions.

This point is critical – once consciousness had evolved, representations of socially relevant perceptions (e.g. a particular person) could be 'evaluated' by correlating a perception with subsequent changes in body state (e.g. fear after seeing that particular person). Thus a particular person would be evaluated as 'fear-provoking'. Social events often lead to emotional responses and adaptive behaviour – and fear of a particular person may lead to avoidance without awareness of the process. However, in a conscious animal, cognitive representations of both the social event and the resulting emotion can interact in working memory, and we can become aware that we fear a particular person because the juxtaposition has occurred in working memory.

This perceptual–emotional interaction creates the potential for *new kinds* of cognitive representation – representations consisting of information from both the senses and the body. It is an accidental by-product of convergence in working memory that these new kinds of perceptual–emotional representation are able to become the subject of awareness. Awareness of inner body states is not the

primary role of consciousness – rather it is an epiphenomenon of the fact that convergence is attained in working
memory, because that is just the way things happened to
evolve. If, in an alternative history, internal and external
information converged in a different part of the brain to
WM, then presumably we would not be aware of body
states – and we would not therefore be 'conscious'.

It is probable that consciousness is crucially dependent
upon neural circuits located in the prefrontal cerebral
cortex of humans, which is the most recently evolved part
of the human brain. The dorsolateral (DL) prefrontal cortex
– the upper outer lobes of the front of the brain – is likely to
be the site of working memory in humans. Indeed, it is
perhaps specifically the DL frontal cortex of the *dominant*
(language-containing) hemisphere. Working memory
probably functions by having arrays of 'delay neurones' that
are capable of remaining active for longer than most
neurones, and by arranging these in a hierarchical pattern.
Information from different perceptual inputs which is fed
into working memory at the posterior part of the DL
prefrontal cortex can become integrated as it converges
towards the upper levels of the hierarchy. Thus, in most
people, working memory is probably located in the large
dome of brain above the left eye and extending about one
third of the way back – and the further forward one goes,
the more integrated the information becomes and the
'higher' the level of processing.

I suggest that body-state representations are constructed
in the parietal lobe of the non-dominant (usually right)
cortex, so that information on the state of the body
converges on the non-dominant parietal lobe, is interpreted
for its emotional importance, and behaviours are initiated
that are appropriate to this information – the whole process
occurring without any need for conscious awareness. The
parietal region seems to be necessary for interpretation of
the biological meaning of body-state feedback in terms of
relevance to behaviour.

In other words, the parietal region appears to conceptualise feedback in terms of a continuously updated body
image, and the continual updating of this image is neces-

sary to the experience of emotions. Without the relevant parietal region, body states would not be interpretable. Destruction of the right-sided parietal region (e.g. by a stroke or a traumatic brain injury) will destroy the body-image representation, and the ability to determine what is body and what is not will be lost. In the common phenomenon of 'neglect' or anosognosia, a person with a non-dominant parietal lesion may lose their awareness of the opposite side of their body. While they are actually looking at their left hand, they may be able to comprehend that it is indeed a part of their body. However, when they are not observing the hand and rely solely on internal information, this awareness is lost – presumably the hand is omitted from their body image – and they may neglect to move or care for the left hand, and may even deny that it belongs to them, or feel that it is an alien hand. This emphasises the extent to which humans depend on an internal representation of their body state in order to monitor and control the body.

Continually updated body-state representations are projected from the right parietal lobe, across the fibres of the corpus callosum that link the two sides of the brain, and to the left dorsolateral prefrontal lobe. Just as destruction to the non-dominant parietal prevents the body-state information from being constructed into a body image, so any lesion to the fibres that cross the corpus callosum or penetrate the prefrontal lobe will prevent body-image representations reaching WM. Since the somatic marker mechanism (SMM) loses emotional input, and perceptions cannot be evaluated by reference to the body states (emotions) that they evoke, lesions to the non-dominant parietal or to the corpus callosum are associated with impaired social intelligence. For example, severing the corpus callosum as a treatment for epilepsy or severing the horizontal connections between the prefrontal region of the cortex and the rest of the brain (as in certain types of 'leucotomy') will both severely impair social intelligence – consistent with the assumption that social intelligence needs emotional information (i.e. body states) in order to perform its function. A patient with a right-sided stroke will often deny that they have any disability, and their social judgement is very poor. Similarly, 'split-brain' patients with a surgically severed corpus callosum apparently cannot cope with employment that requires the exercise of planning and judgement, and their social interactions are impaired.

Why can we be aware of body states?

Why should animals such as humans have evolved to become aware of body states? One answer to this question is that awareness of body states was adaptive, enabling evaluation of social information by emotions, and this gave the conscious animal competitive advantages in the social arena by enabling *strategic* social intelligence. However, it is not the awareness of body states that is adaptive in itself – rather, we are aware of our body states as an accidental by-product of the fact that they are juxtaposed with percep-tions in working memory. The ability to 'introspect' and become aware of our internal milieu (e.g. heartbeat, abdom-inal sensations, tiredness, etc.) does not *itself* have an adaptive function.

It is often stated that the things that consciousness does could be achieved equally well or better without conscious-ness – for example, by a 'zombie'. Theorists arguing along this line either suggest that consciousness is non-adaptive – an accidental by-product of something else – or they argue that it is a mechanism necessary for the solution of some particular adaptive problem that can *only* be solved by consciousness, or at least a problem for which conscious-ness provides the simplest or most efficient engineering solution.

However, this is a non-biological and potentially misleading approach to understanding adaptive function. There are many theoretical potential solutions to any specific behavioural problem. The actual solution reached by natural selection is seldom the simplest or most efficient engineering solution. This is because contingent historical factors constrain the possible directions that natural selection can take, each evolutionary step must be an incremental improvement on what went before, and furthermore the genetic mutations upon which adaptations are built are random and undirected. In the case of consciousness, constraints such as the previously existing structure of the brain are critical in determining the range of possibilities for subsequent evolution.

Consciousness is *sufficient* to perform its adaptive function, but not *necessary*

The fact that a cognitive task could *in principle* be performed without consciousness is irrelevant to the adaptive argument. Even if the task could be performed more simply and efficiently by other methods, the only thing that matters is what, as a matter of historical fact, was the actual solution arrived at by natural selection.

Consciousness is therefore required to be sufficient, but not necessary, for the performance of the task which it is evoked to explain – just as legs are sufficient but not necessary for locomotion. Wheels would also do the job. The 'ultimate' reason why humans locomote by legs rather than wheels is a matter of contingent historical constraints rather than, say, mechanical effectiveness or engineering simplicity. Whatever the relative functional pros and cons of wheels *versus* legs, humans just happen to have evolved from ancestors with legs – wheels were not an option. Similarly, consciousness working by awareness of body states was not the only way of integrating emotions and social perceptions, and the task could *in principle* (i.e. under different constraints) have been done without awareness.

To recapitulate, in principle humans would not need to be aware of body states in order to integrate body-state information with perceptual information. If our evolutionary history had taken a different path, then integration *might* have been achieved in brain regions where cognitive processing did not reach awareness. However, by the 'accidents' of evolutionary history, working memory happened to be the place where emotions and perceptions were brought together. Thus human awareness of emotions is a consequence of contingent evolutionary factors – it is not a formally necessary aspect of strategic social intelligence, and in this sense its *mechanism* is accidental. At the same time, the awareness of emotions does not in its own right confer an adaptive advantage – it is only the convergence of emotions with social perceptions in working memory that is adaptive. Its mechanism will now be explored.

The somatic marker mechanism

Emotions and feelings

According to Damasio, the primary evolutionary function of the animal brain was to serve as an integrative centre to monitor, co-ordinate and regulate the 'inner world' of a complex organism. Therefore the human brain, like the brains of other complex animals, receives on-line, continuously updated representations of the state of the body. These representations are mostly derived from sensory autonomic nerves from the inner organs and somatic nerves from muscles and skin, modified by hormonal chemical messages. They comprise the afferent or feedback arm of a feedback and control mechanism for monitoring, integrating and modulating the current 'state of the organism' – internal viscera, skin, muscle, connective tissue, joints, blood chemistry, and so on.

It seems likely that there is a region of the parietal lobe in the 'non-dominant' hemisphere of the cerebral cortex (i.e. the side that does not have the language specialisation – usually the right-hand side) that is responsible for integrating information from body-state feedback to create a continually updated representation of the body state. If this region is destroyed (e.g. when someone has a stroke affecting the right parietal lobe) then a phenomenon termed 'neglect' or anosognosia is exhibited, in which the affected person becomes unaware of all or part of the left side of the body and visual field, i.e. that part controlled by the right cerebral hemisphere.

'Feelings' occur when body-state representations in working memory indicate a change in body state in response to a change in the environment. Thus consciousness uses feedback concerning body states in order to *evaluate* perceptual inputs, by juxtaposing feelings with the perceptions that have preceded them. In other words, changes in the *soma* (body) are used to *mark* perceptions in working memory. Perceptual–emotional representations are formed – representations which encode information about both perceptual information and the body state that occurred in response to it. We might imagine a visual perception of an aggressive male as one representation and the emotion of terror as another – both active in working memory at the same time. The SMM will combine these two representations to create a single representation (aggressive male – fear) which when it is activated in working memory will elicit both recognition of the perception and replaying of the emotion.

Perceptual–emotional representations evolved in order to deal with *social* situations in particular – consciousness is adapted to function as an aspect of social intelligence. In summary, the somatic marker mechanism (SMM) evolved in order to evaluate social information and enable strategic social intelligence.

Theory of mind and the somatic marker mechanism

The somatic marker mechanism is a vital aspect of the so-called *theory-of-mind mechanism* (ToMM), although (I shall argue) the full theory-of-mind ability requires language as well as the SMM.

Theory of mind has been proposed as a cognitive mechanism by which overt behaviour is interpreted in the light of inferred mental attributes. In other words, an animal with the ToMM is able to make a 'theory' about the contents of another animal's mind. This is the ability that Baron-Cohen has termed 'mind-reading'. The ability is termed a 'theory' of mind mechanism, because the attribution of the mental contents of another animal is based on inference. Obviously animals do not have *direct* access to the contents of each other's minds, and every inference is in this sense a 'theory'. From observation of behaviour and context I may draw the conclusion that someone is angry, but I don't know for sure that the person feels anger. This is a theory designed to account for the situation and predict the future outcomes, and humans are good enough at this kind of mind-reading for loss of the ability (as in autism) to be a severe handicap.

In an animal with a ToMM, the primary interpretative inference is 'mentalistic', and *overt* behaviour is understood in the context of ascribed motivations, dispositions and intentions. For example, we infer the meaning of a *smile* by reference to a person's state of mind – the smile could be understood as one of sympathy, of shared delight, of ingratiating deception, or perhaps a superior sneer, according to our understanding of the smiler's state of mind. By contrast, it is assumed that most animals – lacking a ToMM – infer the meaning of behaviour directly from overt behavioural cues. To such an animal a smile is unambiguously a smile – an expression having a single meaning.

The selection pressure which led to the evolution of theory of mind was probably the potential ambiguity of social cues when overt behaviour is ambiguous (e.g. when behaviour is complex, rapidly changing, or deceptive). When behavioural cues are ambiguous, interpretation of a given cue becomes dependent on inferences concerning intentions, dispositions and relationships.

For example, the approach of another human is ambiguous – it may have several meanings, some hostile and some friendly. In the interpretative sequence 'That man is angry, and approaching me – therefore I must get ready to fight', the mentalistic ascription of anger is logically prior to the interpretation of overt behavioural cues. If the ascription of disposition were to be changed from 'angry' to 'happy', then even when the immediately perceived cues are identical, the inferred meaning of the overt behaviour 'approaching me' (and the implications for an adaptive response) would also change.

As a plausible example, in chimpanzees the approach of a male stranger might evoke fear – the physiological state of arousal in preparedness for 'fight or flight'. This response comprises a characteristic physiological state. Cognitive representations of changing body state are continually constructed in the brain from feedback from the afferent nerves, chemoreceptors and other inputs, probably converging and being integrated in the right-sided parietal lobe. So *emotions* are created in this way, using feedback from the body.

In an animal that lacks a somatic marker mechanism, such cognitive representations of the changing body state may affect behaviour – so that the emotion of fear might provoke involuntary flight. However, in an animal with a somatic marker mechanism, a cognitive representation of this changing body state may be projected forward into the prefrontal cortex and the region which performs the working memory function. In working memory the body state representation that is the emotion of fear becomes accessible to awareness as a conscious *feeling* of fear. The cognitive representation of 'fear' may then be used as a somatic marker when sustained in working memory in temporal juxtaposition to the perceptual representation of the male stranger's identity.

The juxtaposition of the somatic marker for fear with the stranger's identity that evoked it creates a novel cognitive representation incorporating what is, in effect, the *disposition* of that individual – this stranger is disposed to be violent. Although it does not specifically make reference to the mind, this is a theory-of-mind inference – an inference that the stranger is of aggressive intent. The combined perceptual–emotional representation is implicitly one of 'that fear-evoking stranger' (i.e. aggression and hostility are attributed as a 'theory' of the stranger's mental contents). The combined representation can be stored in long-term memory, and when recalled to working memory it will be capable of re-evoking individual identity (perception) and simultaneously re-enacting the linked body state of fear (emotion) as a change in body state.

The ventromedial (lower middle) prefrontal cortex appears to be necessary for the interaction of body-state representations with working memory that enables consciousness. What possibly happens is that working memory in the upper outer (DL) frontal lobe sends a message down through the inner-middle (VM) frontal lobe to deeper structures called the *basal ganglia*, which then evoke the appropriate emotional state in the rest of the body. In patients who have suffered damage to either the ventromedial prefrontal cortex or the basal ganglia, this damage can prevent the expression of secondary emotional states in response to cognitive modelling. The assumption is that upper-outer frontal, inner-middle frontal and basal ganglia form links in a chain that produce emotion in response to cognitive representations in working memory. If this chain is broken, then we would no longer be able to experience fear as a result of *imagining* frightening events, although we would still experience fear in response to actual frightening events. We would no longer enact the emotion of fear when thinking about a tiger attack, although a real-life tiger attack would still produce arousal and flight.

Internal modelling of behaviour by the somatic marker mechanism

The somatic marker mechanism is a system for internally modelling social behaviour and its emotional consequences. The possibility of creating a combined perceptual–emotional representation means that social relationships can be variously combined and sequenced in working memory, and the consequences of this deployment can be evaluated by re-experiencing the enacted emotional body state as gratifying or aversive.

For instance, in an ancestral situation, perhaps the representation of my aggressive and lustful male cousin is recalled from long-term memory along with a representation of my beautiful but gullible daughter, and these two representations are juxtaposed in working memory. Their interaction will perhaps lead to the enactment of an aversive emotion of anxiety which would suggest that bringing these two people together in real life should only be done with caution. Alternatively, modelling the possible outcome of my having a fight with this male cousin might lead to the enactment of a pleasurable sensation, which would encourage me to challenge this potentially dangerous character.

These examples are simplified, but they perhaps communicate the idea that because of the somatic marker mechanism, secondary emotions will accompany the interaction of representations in working memory, and these emotions serve as a guide to interpreting the past and planning future social behaviours. These emotions enacted in response to imagined scenarios are presumed to influence our choice of future action. At the simplest level, we are more likely to pursue a course of action which, when played out by the somatic marker mechanism, leads to a gratifying outcome than we are to pursue a course of action that leads to an aversive outcome. This is what I mean by *strategic* social intelligence – it involves the ability to decide which of various alternative strategies to pursue on the basis of modelling social interactions and evaluating them by the brain sensing how the predicted outcome *feels* to us as emotions are enacted in our bodies.

Somatic marking is therefore the actual mechanism of theory of mind, and in this sense the somatic marker mechanism is the basis of 'mind-reading' – it is a mechanism for inferring what are *de facto* intentions, motivations and dispositions. None the less, the somatic marker mechanism could be regarded as almost the *reciprocal* of the common cognitive conceptualisation of the theory-of-mind mechanism. For example, hostility would not be represented directly as the hostile contents of another's mind, but instead as the reciprocal attribution of the feeling of 'fear'. A 'hostile' male stranger would actually be represented by the somatic marker mechanism as a 'fear-evoking' male stranger – an identity 'marked' by an emotion – with the inference that if we feel fear, then he is probably hostile.

Tactical and strategic social intelligence

The behaviour of Damasio's patients with damage to the system that enacts secondary emotions is characterised by exactly this kind of poor judgement in interpreting and planning social behaviours, and other complex behaviours such as business decisions and gambling. The concept of strategic social intelligence requires further elucidation, both here and elsewhere. Strategy can be contrasted with tactics – strategy being long-term, and tactics being concerned with the here and now; strategy being concerned with general plans, and tactics being a matter of immediate responses.

It is presumed that the somatic marker mechanism is not used in *tactical* social interactions, since the demand for high-speed responsivity dictates that behaviours are elicited by directly reading off the meaning of overt behavioural cues. Modelling in working memory occurs over a time scale of hundreds or thousands of milliseconds, and deploying emotions in the body by the autonomic nervous system and hormonal regulation occurs over an even slower time scale of seconds or minutes. When engaged in face-to-face argument or flirtation, facial expression, gesture and language must all be minutely and rapidly responsive to the situation (over a time scale that is tens or hundreds of times more rapid than working memory), and this kind of tactical social intelligence occurs by 'instinctive' and unconscious mechanisms. However, planned and reflective social interactions – *strategic* social intelligence – depend upon mental modelling.

Of course, strategic and tactical social intelligence will interact. In conscious animals, mentalistic ascriptions of the theory-of-mind type form a 'mind-set', in place in advance of tactical interactions. Each mind-set establishes a tendency for interpretation of cues. Thus if we fear an individual on the basis of strategic modelling of their intentions, then we will tend to interpret tactical behavioural cues in the light of their being hostile. For instance, if you have decided that our lustful cousin intends to seduce your daughter, then his 'tactical' here-and-now behaviour will be interpreted in the light of that assumption. You will therefore interact in a suspicious and cautious manner, and perhaps with a greater tendency towards aggression.

Many behaviours are intrinsically ambiguous, having a variety of possible meanings or being capable of being deployed in a dishonestly manipulative fashion. A gift from the lustful male cousin may be due to generosity or to his intentions with regard to seduction, and which it is will be decided on the basis of strategic modelling of his motivations, intentions and dispositions. This is one plausible interpretation of the chain of events that leads to persecutory delusions – strategic social intelligence creates a mind-set in which we falsely assume hostile intentions in a person. Ambiguous behavioural cues associated with that person are then consistently misinterpreted during tactical interactions, and these misinterpretations serve to reinforce the false belief in hostility.

The evolution of consciousness probably occurred some time before the divergence of the human and chimpanzee lineages, so that modern humans and chimpanzees are both conscious, although human consciousness differs from chimpanzee consciousness, due (mainly) to the addition of abstract symbolic language in humans. Whether consciousness and strategic social intelligence extend further throughout primate species, or to other social mammals (e.g. elephants, dolphins), is a question which would need to be explored in the light of an understanding of the somatic marker mechanism. My hunch is that elephants and dolphins are both conscious, and capable of strategic social intelligence. Time will tell.

Humans are essentially social creatures

The nature of the somatic marker mechanism and the functioning of consciousness mean that the conscious human world is essentially social. This is a matter of common observation. We are aware of people rather than of things, most of our conversation consists of gossip about the doings of other people, our aspirations are usually related to love and status, while our worst fears usually take the form of threats from other humans. Apart from the times when problems of ecological survival are immediate and urgent (e.g. extreme hunger, discomfort or danger), we see the world through social lenses and we pursue social goals.

Kummer has commented on the fact that high status, power and wealth are usually achieved as a result of success in the social realm of human versus human competition, and a person's performance on ecological survival tasks is given much less prestige except in so far as it impinges on this social realm. Thus many of the lowest-status, poorest and most powerless individuals are those doing the 'most important' work of growing and preparing food, providing sanitation, rearing children, building, and so on. At the same time, the rich and famous are often people such as politicians, managers, entertainers or (in other societies) soldiers – that is, people whose relationship to the world of survival is at best indirect.

This is a consequence of the success of social animals in solving problems of survival. When group-living animals have succeeded in developing effective strategies for obtaining food and shelter and repelling predators, then their main source of competition becomes the other members of the group. Thus, although human co-operation is what made us such a successful social animal, at the same time intra-species (between-person) competition characterises the human condition. To use the biological jargon, we are intrinsically both altruistic and agonistic.

Language

On considering the human condition, it is clear that there is much that humans share with other animals – many causes of pleasure and pain, survival or death. However, there is also much about humans that is unique, and of these features probably the most obvious one is language.

It is clear that, in some sense, 'language' is indeed unique to humans, although exactly what it is about language that is unique requires further definition. Many other animals communicate, and a few of them have extremely sophisticated systems of communication. It seems that only humans have evolved a complex, abstract symbolic language which *also* has that feature which is biologically crucial about human communication – human communication is both complex and *capable of displacement*.

Defining 'language' as displacement communication

Displacement refers to the capacity of language to refer to entities and events that are 'displaced' in time or space (i.e. not you or me, not here, or not now). This is the subject matter of much human language – we do not just talk of the here and now, but conversation ranges widely over reminiscence of the past, and hopes and fears for the future. However, although displacement is necessary to allow this, it is not necessarily a part of complex communications systems. For example, the bee dance is an abstract symbolic communication of spatially displaced information, but it occurs in an extremely simple and specific communications system. The dance is capable of transmitting information about where to find nectar in relation to the place of the dance (i.e. displacement to another place), but that is pretty much all the dance can do.

However, displacement in human language is built *on top of* an already extremely sophisticated social communication system which we inherited from our ape and primate ancestors – a system based on facial expression, gesture and a range of sounds. For example, even without language we could talk about 'my brother' and what he is doing at the waterhole. So long as my brother and the waterhole are both present, they can be indicated by gesture, and so long as we restrict ourselves to what is actually happening here and now, then the subject matter can be indicated by further gestures and body language, and our feelings about them indicated by facial expressions and vocalisation. So if my brother was swimming, this could be indicated by pointing at him and the waterhole and miming the swimming. This is how many social animals communicate, and how humans may communicate with other animals (such as dogs), as well as with people who do not have language (such as children), or people with whom we do not share language. However, without some system of displacement we cannot refer to my brother and the waterhole in relation to another time or place, and we could not refer to any person who was not present here and now.

Displacement would inevitably involve some way of symbolising my brother and the waterhole by creating an abstract referent (e.g. this stone is my brother and the leaf is the waterhole, or this gesture, or this word), and by indicating the nature of the relationship between my bother and the waterhole (i.e. swimming – which might be represented by facial expression, gesture and vocalisation for simple concepts). My brother, the waterhole and swimming are a scenario. The act of displacement involves indicating that my brother and the waterhole and the relationship are to be understood as being at another time or place – probably by linking the scenario described above with indicators of another time or place.

Using displacement we might talk of my brother (even though he is not here at present), we might talk of my brother at the waterhole (although the waterhole is not in sight), and we might mention the fact that he is swimming. The scenario is one of my brother swimming at the waterhole, and to perform the displacement we might talk of my brother swimming at the waterhole *last* full moon (in the past), or the conjecture that he may swim at the waterhole *next* full moon (in the future). The scenario is displaced by associating the scenario (brother, waterhole and swimming) with an indicator of a different time or place. Displacement requires merely that we can symbolise the full moon and indicate whether we are referring to the last one or the next one, and that this can be linked to the scenario. My suggestion is that displacement works by establishing such linkages to displace scenarios to other times or places.

Displacement is necessary, but not sufficient, for the definition of language

Displacement is here taken to be the defining feature of *language* as contrasted with communication. Displacement is defining because it is an aspect of communication that could not – even in principle – be replaced by gesture, grunts, facial expression, body language or other non-linguistic communications. Displacement requires symbols, and symbolic communication must already have existed before displacement could have evolved. This implies that symbols can occur without displacement, and that we have inherited a symbolising ability from our primate ancestors. Common chimpanzees and bonobos who have been trained to use large vocabularies of symbols when communicating with humans seem to have considerable abstract symbolic ability. Thus human ancestors already had an ability to symbolise and 'only' needed to evolve the ability to perform displacement.

Displacement is therefore proposed as necessary, although not sufficient, for a communication system to be termed a language. In other words, there is a great deal more to language than just displacement, but without displacement, communication does not count as language. Broadly speaking, chimpanzee ability in communication plus the capability of displacement equals what most people would term a full language – that is, human-type language.

There should be a clear distinction between speech as a

system of communication, and the existence of displacement to constitute language. The highly restrictive definition of only displacement communication as language proper means that most of verbal communication (even in humans) is *not* language, because most communication is in principle potentially replaceable by non-language communication. By this account, most of 'linguistics' is not about language, but about speech. And chimpanzee communication – although it may be very sophisticated, capable of complex instructions, and perhaps even have its own 'grammar' – would *only* be considered a full language if it turns out to be true that chimpanzee communication of social information is indeed displaceable. And the speech of children, or of adults with mental handicap – however subtle a form of here-and-now speech-based communication it may be – would only be considered to constitute a full language if the individuals concerned were able to make functional use of displacement.

However, it is important to point out that the *forms* of displacement, such as the use of words indicative of past and future tense, are not *by themselves* evidence of displacement. For example, it is possible to 'parrot' grammatical forms such as past or future tense without any understanding of how to use them in practice. A demented person may use phrases indicative of false memories or imagined fears for the future, but these are socially (and biologically) non-functional. The test is that full language uses the forms of displacement in a functional way with real-world applicability.

The idea that displacement is a distinctive and defining quality of human language is certainly not currently accepted. At present, many of the formal 'tests' of language ability (e.g. the test 'batteries' used by speech and language researchers) do not function as tests of displacement. For example, when a doctor asks a patient who has had a stroke to name a watch or a pen being presented to them, this does not count as a test of language. Indeed, there are currently no language tests designed specifically to measure the ability to perform displacement. Displacement is not a recognised key variable in language function.

Furthermore, current 'linguistic analysis' is essentially the study of speech or written communication. The discipline of linguistics does not make a distinction between the displacement functions that are unique to language and the use of speech that could, in principle, be replaced by expression and gesture. This highlights the ground that the discipline of linguistics still needs to cover in order to become properly integrated as a biological science.

Why displacement evolved – role and adaptive benefits

The benefits of displacement may seem obvious, since it gives access to knowledge of social events that are remote in space or time, but because displacement does *not* seem to have evolved in other social primate species, such as common chimpanzees, gorillas, orang-utans and baboons, it needs further explanation. If displacement is useful for humans, why has it not (or not obviously) arisen in other primate species?

The assumption that there *is* an adaptive reason why displacement evolved, and that language is not an accidental by-product of some other adaptation, must be justified. The adaptive role of displacement is strongly suggested by the social intelligence perspective which sees language as primarily concerned with the communication of information about human beings and their activities. It should also be borne in mind that human brain tissue is difficult to grow and develop, and is metabolically very expensive to maintain – in other words, brain is a very *costly* tissue. This implies that there must be considerable benefits to offset the costs of substantial neural construction such as was required to support the advanced functions of language.

Almost any level of brain damage to the more recently evolved parts of the cerebral cortex will impair language function. Even when the actual production of grammatical speech is apparently unimpaired (as in non-dominant lobe lesions or frontal lobe lesions), so that the brain-damaged subject can perform purely linguistic tests at a normal level, the actual applicability of language to social situations is almost always impaired. Close study of most patients with any significant degree of brain damage will usually reveal that factors such as appropriateness, prosody (i.e. the rise and fall of intonation) or use of metaphors are impaired – in other words, the social function of language is impaired. Language function certainly appears to depend on brain function, and indeed on sustained function of most of the brain.

The first assumption is that whatever the reason for the evolution of displacement, it is social. This is consistent with the social intelligence assumption that recent human evolution has been driven by social selection pressures. The social assumption reshapes the question about displacement into asking what it was about ancestral human *social organisation* that made displacement so useful, and how these features differed from those of other related ape species which did not evolve displacement as part of their communication systems. This argument is, of course, based on only a few species of primates and (like almost all scientific theorising) it contains some elements of *post hoc* circularity, but this does not mean that the theory is untestable.

Even when methods of testability are not immediately obvious, once a scientific theory has been described in a clear and explicit fashion, it is usually possible to find ways in which to put its novel consequences to the test of observation and experiment.

Constraints on the evolution of displacement language

In a conscious social animal without language (such as a chimpanzee), the somatic marker mechanism enables the modelling of differential social identity together with somatic markers to represent disposition, motivation and intention. The somatic marker mechanism can form combined perceptual–emotional representations (implicitly symbolic) – for example, 'that angry, aggressive male who hates me'. It therefore allows abstract, symbolic thought in which representations can interact and be manipulated. The addition of language to consciousness augments this combined social–emotional representation with further *displacement markers* that are indicative of other times, other places and other people.

The specifically socially adaptive nature of language is supported by evidence from spontaneous language usage (most of which constitutes 'gossip' about the activities of other people), neuroanatomical correlations between regions concerned with language and social intelligence, and temporal and genetic informational constraints on human evolution. At a conservative estimate, only around 5–6 million years have elapsed since divergence of the human lineage from that of chimpanzees, and less than 2000 genes (i.e. less than 2% of the genome) differ between humans and chimpanzees. This amount of DNA has been estimated to contain approximately 35 000 (35K) bits of useful design information, which is not much – certainly not enough to code for something as complex as the whole of the human communication system.

Although the frontal lobe of the brain has expanded substantially since our lineage diverged from that of chimpanzees, the structure of the brain substance itself does not appear to have changed qualitatively. There is no obviously different and new cortical region which has been added to the chimpanzee brain in order to perform the function of language – the human brain just looks like 'more of the same'. It seems as if humans have merely evolved more of the same type of brain substance that was already present in the ancestors we share with chimpanzees – a relatively quick and easy thing to evolve, as it merely requires a few genetic mutations to instruct the body to 'make more of this' and to 'wire it up' in a particular fashion.

These constraints make it likely that the evolution of human linguistic capacity was largely dependent upon pre-established neuroanatomical micro-circuitry, and the evidence with regard to the specifically socially adaptive nature of language means that the neuroanatomical circuitry of language is very probably the system which evolved to subserve social intelligence – in other words, working memory and the somatic marker mechanism. The constraints of limited evolutionary time also imply that the extra computations required for language-processing were relatively simple. The computations are probably of the same kind as those performed in the primate frontal cortex of other species. The difference lies in the connectivity between the computational areas, particularly the addition of extra levels to the hierarchy of convergence and integration.

The extra power of the human brain may be a matter of greater integration. For example, the visual system seems to have evolved by new brain regions sampling more different aspects of the visual information generated by the retina, and bringing together these different aspects in new syntheses to extract more and more information from the same initial signal. In other words, the human brain is pretty much a bigger chimpanzee brain, with most of the extra brain at the front.

Displacement, group size and the sexual division of labour

So why did displacement evolve? If the common chimpanzee is assumed to be closely similar to the human ancestor of five million years ago, and if we assume that the bonobo also evolved from something very like a common chimpanzee, then a plausible scenario can be constructed. Both chimpanzee species exhibit extremely sophisticated 'here-and-now' tactical social communication by facial expression, gesture and verbal signalling, but apparently this communication relates only to individuals and circumstances that are currently present. The question is, under what ecological circumstances might a great ape benefit substantially from an extra ability – the ability to do something more than this and to communicate about individuals who are not present and events that are not taking place now?

My suggestion is that displacement language evolved for two reasons. The first reason is that social groups became sufficiently *large* that unique identities were required to keep track of and refer to individuals. Humans inhabit large social groups compared to chimpanzees, and perhaps this led to an enhanced ability to use abstract symbols to refer to individuals, as it would not always be possible to indicate individuals by gesture. Bonobos seem to have a higher degree of abstract symbolic ability than chimpanzees, which is consistent with the fact that their social groups are much larger. As well as the symbolic ability of chimpanzees and bonobos that have been trained to use abstract geometrical shapes to communicate with humans, examples of symbol use have been recorded in natural conditions – for example, the young bonobo that used a log of wood as a 'doll' to play with exactly as if it were a baby, or the way in which bonobos communicate the need to move on to a new camp by dragging a large branch around the troop and showing it to each member, the branch apparently serving as a symbol (presumably learned) of the need to move.

However, for displacement to be useful, as well as a large group size it may also be necessary that the group splits up for significant periods before being reunited. So the second selection pressure favouring displacement would be *division of labour* – tasks dividing the group for significant but temporary periods. Given that language (it is assumed) evolved for the communication of information about other people, splitting of the larger group into smaller groups for significant periods would mean that communication of information about other members of the group who were *not present* would require displacement. The advantage of this is that individuals and their behaviours can be evaluated in their absence – for example, information could be gathered concerning the suitability of a potential mate or the attributes of a rival.

Humans under ancestral conditions exhibited exactly such a division of labour. Ancestral groups were nomadic foragers, and these groups would have split up frequently and for hours or even days at a time, due to the sexual division of labour – men going off to hunt while the women remained near the camp, gathering vegetable food and looking after the children. My idea is that this splitting up of the troop would have provided a strong selection pressure to favour those people who could talk about others even while they were not present, and 'gossip' in order to understand their personality, interpret their past behaviours and predict their next moves.

For instance, one plausible scenario is that displacement language may have evolved initially *among women* for exchanging information about the absent men, in order to evaluate potential mates and discover more about the behaviour of the males of the family. Females could exchange knowledge (which might, of course, be biased or deceptive) concerning the absent males. Men are often the topic of conversation among women under such circumstances today. By contrast, while displacement would certainly enhance the planning of hunting in principle, such planning is clearly not essential to the activity of hunting. Very many animals, including common chimpanzees, hunt effectively in groups without the need for displacement language, and hunting does not appear to be a selection pressure for displacement ability. Moreover, men who are hunting are often quiet and speak little to one another.

Thus this scenario suggests that displacement language initially evolved *primarily* to benefit women in exchanging information about men who were away hunting, but this language ability was also inherited by men, as most inherited traits are shared and displacement would also have benefited men, albeit in a secondary fashion. This speculation fits contemporary evidence of higher-level linguistic ability ('verbal intelligence') in women, a high frequency of spontaneous language use among groups of women, and the observation that the subject matter of private woman-to-woman conversations is often focused on the subject of men.

I find the story both plausible and attractive, but inconclusive. It could be tested by further study of communication and language use in chimpanzees, and especially bonobos. Although bonobos do not show sexual division of labour, their groups are large (consisting of many dozens of individuals), and since bonobos live in the jungle they would not be able to keep all group members under observation. This would be a selection pressure for some degree of displacement, and it might explain the greater linguistic ability of bonobos compared with common chimpanzees.

Displacement in working memory depends on sufficient spatial capacity for complex representations

The radical view put forward here is that there are no recently evolved specialised 'language centres' in the brain, but that instead displacement language has been made possible by a *quantitative* expansion of the functional capability of working memory, on top of the already evolved and pre-existing somatic marker mechanism.

This view is in contradiction to a vast amount of linguistic, neurological and evolutionary speculation which is based on a different conceptualisation of language (a conceptualisation which does not, for example, define displacement as the crux of language, and which does not clearly differentiate language from speech). However, when the concept of language is built up in this stepwise and evolutionary fashion, by considering the somatic marker mechanism assumed to be present in chimpanzees and bonobos and adding the capacity of displacement, it then becomes plausible that the evolution of language may be a much simpler and more straightforward matter than is usually believed.

The basic, underlying principle of displacement of socially relevant information could be the interaction of representations created by the somatic marker mechanism, with further markers for displacement. What is envisaged is that, for example, a representation such as 'aggressive male cousin' is a combined perceptual–emotional representation comprising (at least) two representations that have been combined in working memory. There is a representation of the perception of a specific person (the male cousin) and a representation of the associated emotional state from which we infer that the male cousin is aggressive. To displace the representation of aggressive male cousin requires *nothing more* than to create an association with a further symbolic marker which represents another time or another place.

Thus this entity of 'aggressive male cousin' contains both perceptual information on individual identity and the information to trigger a specific emotional response. This perceptual–emotional representation may be associated with a symbolic marker that represents (for example) a temporal displacement such as 'tomorrow morning', or a spatial displacement such as 'waterhole', or a symbol for another person (including the emotional response) such as 'my younger sister'. The process is one of incremental expansion and association of information in working memory, whereby representations are 'superimposed' and loaded with more and more information – both perceptual and emotional.

A large-capacity working memory can therefore create very complex representations, and these representations can enable displacement, or indeed some other extra complexity of information. Incremental expansion of working memory over an evolutionary time scale is biologically plausible, and would enable progressively more of these iterative associations to be accumulated within the capacity of working memory.

Limits of working memory

What are the limits of working memory? What defines how much it can carry? As working memory is essentially an anatomical space where representations (in the form of three-dimensional patterns of neural activity) are *sustained*, then the major constraints on the capacity of working memory are set by the complexity of representations that may be sustained, and by the duration for which representations may be sustained. In other words, the size of working memory is defined by the *capacity* of WM (how complex a representation it can accommodate) and by the *time span* of WM (how long the representations can be sustained).

Capacity is probably constrained by the size of the part of the brain devoted to WM (the more neurones there are in WM, the greater the complexity of representation it can enact). Time span probably constrains the number of representations that may be kept active simultaneously – along the lines of 'Miller's magic number' (known to all psychology undergraduates), which suggests that a maximum of 5–9 items can be sequentially loaded and retained in working memory at one time. The exact number is less important than the fact that there is some such temporal limit on the time span over which an item can be kept active in WM.

In evolutionary history, the capacity and time span of working memory would presumably have varied between species according to evolutionary constraints, with some species being able to retain items over a longer time span, and some able to enact larger and more complex representations than others. Evidence from maze tasks suggests that humans and rats do not differ substantially in the time span of working memory, and it is likely that the very great size of the dorsolateral prefrontal cortex implies that the special thing about human working memory is the size and complexity of representations that it is capable of sustaining (rather than a particularly large capacity for sequential loading with items). This is speculative, but it seems plausible that the large volume of the anatomical substrate of human memory evolved in order to allow complex (and hence large-volume) cognitive representations to be enacted.

According to current evidence, it seems that the working memory of a common chimpanzee is insufficient to support the displacement of social information, although it is possible that specific individual chimpanzees with exceptionally large WM capacity may be able to perform displacement. It may also be that chimpanzees can perform displacement on tasks which are computationally simpler than social intelligence. As suggested by the work of Sue Savage Rumbaugh, bonobos may be much closer to possessing a human-like language ability, which implies that they should have a larger-capacity WM than the common chimpanzee. Clearly these questions would require specific exploration.

However, the assumption here is that the chimpanzee WM has the same nature and functional capability as the human WM – and that the only important structural difference relates to size. The idea is that the evolution of the very large human prefrontal cortex was driven by the advantages of expanding WM, and the primary function that was served by the expansion of WM was displacement language – that is, the ability to form complex associations not just of social identity and emotion, but also markers of other times and places. Such representations containing information about people, emotional reactions to these people and also markers of other places and/or times would presumably be highly complex and large, requiring a greater capacity from WM.

It should also be emphasised that the neural substrate for displacement is not specific to displacement. The expansion of WM over human evolutionary history has a very wide range of other consequences, since it enables greatly increased complexity of all types of cognitive modelling – an increase in what many people would consider to be 'general intelligence'.

Expanded WM also enables other types of complex grammatical construction such as representing contingency, and performing many layers of embedding of clauses.

In summary, the assertion is that the selection pressure for the expansion of WM capacity occurred in order to enable displacement of language – this was its selective driving force – and therefore that enabling displacement is the *adaptive* consequence of expanded WM. The other consequences of expanded WM capacity, such as many aspects of 'general intelligence', although perhaps more obvious under modern conditions, are epiphenomenal by-products when viewed from an evolutionary perspective.

Some consequences and predictions

To put it crudely but reasonably accurately, a human brain may be pretty much *a chimpanzee brain with a larger working memory* (plus some motor and auditory specialisations to enable speech). The larger size of human working memory means that larger and more complex patterns of nerve activation (cognitive representations) can be accommodated, and these representations can become so complex as to include information on social identity, emotion and displacement.

General-purpose human intelligence, as applied to the vast range of cultural activity, is an accidental consequence of the adaptive benefits of social intelligence, especially the somatic marker mechanism and the need to displace social information. The enhanced human ability to symbolise may also be a consequence of expanded working memory, so that very complex representations can then be further linked to abstract perceptual entities (such as words).

Presumably symbolisation is made possible by the association of representations that occur in working memory. A perceptual representation interacts with an emotional representation to form a bridging representation that links both. Thus the bonobo links the perceptual representation of a baby with a particular baby-sized piece of wood, or it links the need to move camp with the dragging of a branch. The symbol also links the relevant emotions (evoked by a real baby, or a need to move) to the symbolic use of a particular shape and size of wood. With the doll, a specific piece of wood acts to trigger a mental representation which both recalls a baby and evokes the emotions appropriate to a baby. The wood is an effective symbol of the baby because it stands for both identity and emotion.

Enhancing chimpanzee working memory

This relatively simple scheme seems to include, in outline, many of the features that a biological description of language would require. One way to test it would be somehow to increase the working memory of a chimpanzee, and to see whether this brought its communication ability towards that of humans. It is possible that this amplification of working memory is exactly what has been achieved by teaching chimpanzees the use of visual symbols on a board – each symbol is a convenient 'chunk' of the perceptual features of that to which it refers. Each symbol is 'stored' on a board for reference, which leaves more of the chimpanzee working memory free to manipulate and integrate other representations. Symbol boards can be regarded as an indirect method for amplifying chimpanzee working memory, rather as humans amplify working memory by writing or using counters to calculate.

Certainly it seems that the better a common chimpanzee or bonobo can master a symbol board, the more human-like their language becomes, and it does not seem too unlikely that Doctor Doolittle's desire to 'talk to the animals' may have been achieved by Sue Savage Rumbaugh and her bonobos.

Humans with low-capacity working memory may lack language (i.e. lack displacement)

If displacement language depends on working memory in a quantitative fashion, then this has several other testable consequences. Humans who have WM capacity below a critical threshold, perhaps due to brain trauma, disease, congenital brain damage or other forms of intellectual handicap, would be expected to display reduced WM capacity and also to lack displacement language, *even when* they have speech and the ability to communicate theory-of-mind information. Once again it is important to emphasise the difference between speech and language.

Thus, for example, the prediction is that mentally handi-capped individuals with Williams' syndrome, who are supposed to have remarkable social and 'linguistic' abilities, would be found on specific examination to lack the ability to perform functionally effective displacement with language. Displacement is not, of course, merely a matter of being able to use the appropriate grammatical forms such as 'tense' – that could be achieved by merely 'parroting' (i.e. repeating without understanding forms heard elsewhere). However, the displacement language must also be adaptive, appropriate to the social situation, and refer to real-world events.

The social structure of language

The somatic marker mechanism is not restricted to social information, because working memory is not restricted to social information (which is not a distinct module, but is composed of projections from a wide variety of processed perceptual data as well as information on body states). This means that these associations are not confined to social, temporal and spatial information, but may be used to relate any kind of associations. Thus although the adaptive function of consciousness is specific to social intelligence, the mechanisms are general-purpose, and non-social information can use the somatic marker mechanism processes as an accidental by-product of brain connectivity.

Language, by its location in working memory, serves as a 'translation' device by which non-social domains of knowledge can gain access to the cognitive apparatus that evolved to deal with social intelligence. Working memory is an association mechanism, and any entities that can be deployed in WM can be associated with one another. Presumably this is why humans can use their social intelligence to reason about non-social matters such as technology and natural history, by using the somatic marker mechanism in an expanded-capacity working memory.

In effect, humans use social intelligence as a system for generating *analogies*, so that different classes of proposition are processed as if they were social problems. Much of high-level human intelligence can be considered as analogical –

a system in which the somatic marker mechanism works by 'anthropomorphising' non-social topics as if they were stories about intentional agents. I have discussed this further in the chapter on creativity.

This capacity to 'over-learn' new topics on to the somatic marker evaluation system of social intelligence has proved to be the crucial factor in the development of 'symbolic' human culture.

Language and the human condition

This book is only about language in so far as language is a major element in human nature – language is an aspect of what Bronowski called 'human specificity'. Language is a major part of what makes humans distinctive.

The prevailing view of the nature and structure of language is dominated by the assumption that language is a general-purpose specialisation. By contrast, the social theory of language assumes that language evolved for the purpose of communicating social information ('gossiping', as Dunbar terms it). The concept of displacement communication is an incomplete evolutionary and neuroscientific account of full language. In particular, the above scheme distinguishes language from speech, and says nothing about the anatomical, motor and perceptual specialisations necessary for verbal communication of language. However, the above view assumes that most of what linguists call 'language' is not biologically distinct from other forms of verbal and gestural communication. Only displacement language is biologically distinct from other forms of here-and-now communication.

This view also overturns the idea of traditionally defined 'language areas'. Brain areas such as Broca's and Wernicke's areas are actually concerned with *speech* – that is, with verbal communication rather than language. For example, Broca's area is concerned with fine control of motor systems (including those involved in the articulation of speech), while Wernicke's area is probably concerned with specialisations of the sense of hearing and verbal monitoring that evolved along with the evolution of verbal communication.

The remarkable sureness and rapidity of human language acquisition are seen as a consequence of the human drive to communicate, combined with the gradual maturation of the central nervous system. There is no evolved 'language-acquisition device' which makes us learn language. The drive to communicate is based on our fundamental nature as social animals, and the immediate advantages a child obtains from his or her ability to communicate social information. Normal children communicate as soon as the maturity of the nervous system allows them to do so, and it is the maturation of the nervous system which times the stages of linguistic development. Common observation shows that in a social milieu a child wants to communicate social information, and tries to talk because it is so useful in that social environment. Learning to talk happens when the physical apparatus of speech is mature, and when the working memory capacity has grown to a sufficient size. Displacement is the last major attribute of language to occur in a normal developing child (at about the time when myelinisation of the central nervous system is complete), and displacement presumably occurs when working memory is large enough to deploy the complex representations which displacement requires.

The social theory of consciousness and language also makes some predictions about the structure of language – its grammar. It predicts that much of the structure of language derives from social intelligence – in other words, from the structure and operation of the somatic marker mechanism. It is possible that social entities (intentional agents such as persons) and the nature of social interactions (as represented by the somatic marker mechanism) might constitute some of the fundamental categories of language. These speculations are beyond the scope of this book, but will be pursued elsewhere.

The crucial point about the dependence of distinctively human intelligence on the somatic marker mechanism is that, because it is based on social categories and driven by social motivations, even our abstract thought world is saturated with emotions, preferences and aversions, pleasures and pain. At a deep level, this is why humans are able to care about that accidental and artificial product of human invention which we call culture.

Human creativity and the *Col-oh-nell Flastratus* phenomenon

Creativity and culture

At first sight, creativity appears to be distinctive to humans, although the more we discover about chimpanzees, the more creative they seem to be. Both common chimpanzees and bonobos are able to innovate and transmit innovations to such an extent that each group could be described as possessing a 'culture'. Wrangham and Peterson have listed the contents of such a culture, which include the use of tools (termite probes, sponges, etc.) and protective 'clothing' (e.g. 'slippers' and 'umbrellas' made of leaves).

If this is culture at its simplest, the following section focuses on the opposite extreme – creativity at its highest levels, and the special human satisfactions that are derived from creative activity.

A dream

Some years ago I had a bizarre dream in which I was vouchsafed a secret which would ensure my wealth and success. I will now share the secret. It was the title for a comic novel – a title so loaded with humorous potential, so funny even in its own right, that it would (I was assured) guarantee classic status for any book to which it was attached. The title was *Oh Colonel Flastratus!* The important factors about this title were twofold. First, the word 'Colonel' should be spelled conventionally but pronounced in three syllables – Col-oh-nell. Somehow this had to be communicated to the potential audience through advertising. Secondly, the exclamation mark at the end was vital in order to convey the correct tone of exasperation.

The distinctive feature about my dream was not its silliness but that for several minutes, at least, the event possessed a quality of profound significance. On awakening, I wrote down the title and puzzled over its meaning and consequences. Quite abruptly it dawned on me that, whatever its numinous quality, the objective content of my experience was nil. The only 'funny' thing about *Oh Colonel Flastratus!* was the surrealist absurdity of my having attached significance to it.

However, if it had not been for this absurdity, my dream had all the subjective hallmarks of a transcendental or mystical episode. Perhaps if the title had possessed more conventionally spiritual connotations, or if my own sense of the ridiculous had been less acute, or if I had lived in a different society, I would indeed have placed a religious interpretation on the dream. The experience might have seemed like a message from the gods, or enlightenment. If it caught on, we might have had a *Colonel Flastratus* cult on our hands.

Peak experiences

Such experiences are not uncommon. The psychologist Abraham Maslow wrote extensively on the subject in the middle of this century. He labelled the phenomena 'peak experiences' (PEs). Peak experiences are those moments, lasting from seconds to minutes, during which we feel the highest levels of happiness, harmony and possibility. They range in degree from intensifications of everyday pleasure to apparently 'supernatural' episodes of enhanced consciousness which feel qualitatively distinct from, and superior to, normal experience.

Some people regard PEs as pointing the way towards what ought to be the norm in a truly healthy, ideal human life. By this account, normal everyday life is a disease state during which we function at a lower level – firing on three cylinders, as it were. Everyday life is semi-human, and only during peak experiences are we fully awake, alert, aware, conscious and alive. According to this view, PEs are to be valued as providing a privileged insight into 'reality'. Because they represent a *higher* state of consciousness, knowledge obtained in this state has greater validity than the insights of the normal, suboptimal level of consciousness associated with mundane existence. Certainly peak experiences constitute some of the most memorable and subjectively significant events in life.

I do not go along with the idea that peak experiences are a window on to a transcendental reality (because I do not believe there is such a thing), nor do I consider that they constitute a pathway to a higher 'evolutionary' state (because I do not recognise any other significant creative evolutionary process than the very slow workings of natural selection). Nevertheless, there seems to be something worth pursuing in the idea that PEs are of special significance. Certainly, they do not strike at random – they are associated with particular circumstances. Furthermore, their occurrence may be associated with a transformation in personal behaviour or goals. The potentially profound *subjective* significance of a peak experience is not open to serious doubt, but the objective validity of the content of that experience is another matter.

Peak experiences in science

The objective significance of a peak experience is a complex matter. The best test of this is a consideration of PEs as they occur in science. Because scientific propositions generated as PEs are susceptible to external validation, they may tell us whether PEs are no more than the *Colonel Flastratus* phenomenon writ large, or whether they might perhaps be indicative of something rather more interesting.

A recent memorable example of a peak experience was reported in an interview on the BBC television programme *Horizon*, in which the mathematician Andrew Wiles described the moment when he solved 'Fermat's last theorem' – a problem that has exercised the minds of the greatest mathematicians for three centuries. After working on the problem for seven years in solitude and secrecy, Wiles announced success – only to find a flaw in the reasoning. Another year of tense and desperate work ensued. Then 'suddenly, totally unexpectedly, I had this incredible revelation... It was so indescribably beautiful; it was so simple and so elegant. I just stared in disbelief for twenty minutes.' As Wiles recounted his peak experience, he became overwhelmed with emotion at the recollection.

This was only a recent instance of overpowering subjective sensations accompanying creative insight. Leo Szilard, the discoverer of the principle of the nuclear 'chain reaction', wrote: 'I remember that I stopped for a red light... As the light changed to green it suddenly occurred to me that if we could find an element... which would emit two neutrons when it absorbed *one* neutron [this] could sustain a nuclear chain reaction'. Thus was discovered the concept which led directly to the development of the atom bomb.

From the original 'eureka' moment of Archimedes in the bath, right through to the other intellectual giants of the twentieth century, the phenomena of scientific creativity display striking similarities. Moreover, peak experiences occur at all levels of achievement, not only the most elevated. There is a special quality attached to the best scientific insights – a sense of crystallisation.

A personal example

I personally have experienced such moments. For example, one evening I had stayed behind to examine some new microscope slides of the human adrenal gland which had been stained to show both the cholinergic and adrenergic nerves. The cholinergic nerves were dark brown, while the adrenergic nerves glowed green under a fluorescent lamp. When I flipped the microscope back and forth between natural light and fluorescent light I suddenly realised that the slender, knobbly green nerves were winding over and around the thick trunks of brown nerves. The two systems were entwined, but the cholinergic nerves were passing through the gland while the adrenergic nerves were releasing their noradrenaline into the substance of the cortex. It suddenly dawned on me that no one had ever seen this before. It was a moment of apparently mystical significance, in that twilit room – I knew something for the first time in human history.

Scientific theories are even more mysterious than experimental discoveries, in that a breakthrough dawns without any insight into the steps by which it was reached. Only afterwards comes an attempt to assemble a rational pathway by which this insight can be justified and defended. In order for the idea potentially to become a part of the body of science – 'reliable' knowledge to be placed before the peer group for debate and critique – propositions must be expressed in a form that will be widely understandable, checkable and usable. This kind of expression may not be an easy task to achieve. It took me more than six months to write the malaise theory of depression as a paper, grappling with expression, and constructing a plausible chain of inference to back up my intuition. It will take even longer to get the idea across to the scientific peer group, constructing a convincing rationale, an enlightening example, a memorable name and an appealing analogy to assist understanding. And it will take even longer to test its scope and validity.

Darwin spent 20 years musing on and gathering evidence for evolution by natural selection before he was stampeded into publication by the fact that Alfred Wallace independently had the same idea (he was also deterred from publication by worry about the controversy which he – accurately – guessed would follow publication). It was a further approximately 100 years before the theory of natural selection was completed by its synthesis with genetics. Einstein had key insights into relativity as a very young man (e.g. when he imagined what it would be like to ride a beam of light), but several years of work were necessary to turn that insight into published science. And Richard Feynman used his diagrams to solve problems of quantum electrodynamic theory for several years without being able to explain what he was doing or why it worked. It required an intervention from his friend Freeman Dyson to indicate to the broader community of physicists just what Feynman was up to. Clearly the insight and its 'translation' into a comprehensible form are two different phenomena, sometimes requiring two different people. WD Hamilton and GC Williams published breakthroughs in evolutionary theory in the early 1960s, but these proved largely incomprehensible until Richard Dawkins re-expressed them and provided the necessary metaphor more than a decade later in his famous book, *The Selfish Gene*.

This is the nature of peak experiences concerned with scientific theory. They are emphatically not self-validating. Even when the insights are of matchless brilliance, their implications must be spelled out and checked. For instance, there was the moment when Francis Crick and his co-workers realised that they had been thinking along the wrong lines about how genes were made into proteins. On the one hand, there was 'the sudden flash of inspiration...that cleared away so many of our difficulties.... When I went to bed...the shining answers stood clearly before me.' On the other hand, Crick knew that 'it would take months and years of work to establish these new ideas'. However, 'We were no longer lost in the jungle.... We could survey the open plain and clearly see the mountains in the distance'.

The nature of the scientific peak experience

The typical insight associated with a peak experience is *integrative* in nature, with the sense of meaningfulness that comes from assembling the right things in the right order to make some kind of sense from them. Jacob Bronowski emphasised that creation exists in finding unity – the likeness and pattern that underlies variety – and that this applies equally to the sciences and the arts. He quotes Samuel Taylor Coleridge: 'beauty is unity in variety'. The moment during which superficial differences crystallise into comprehensible order is the peak experience – it is the 'moment of creation'.

The crystallisation metaphor is in some respects misleading. A theory is much more than a summary and reordering of the facts; a theory postulates that which *lies behind* the facts and generates them. A good theory selects from the facts and points beyond them. Science is structured knowledge, not merely a loose-leaf folder of 'facts'. It is the structure that enables scientific knowledge to be testable.

The peak experience of scientific creativity does not merely constitute a simple, elegant and compelling *arrangement* of data that is already in the mind. It also involves an insight into which of the facts are the important ones, and how they are related to one another by causal processes. A scientific theory involves carving nature into new shapes, and saying it is *this* that matters rather than that; and *these* processes rather than those.

Thus as well as integration of previous knowledge, the PE is typified by a sense of possibility. It can be conceptualised as a point of stillness, where an understanding of the past and the potential of the future intersect, so that the PE is a reaching of conclusions which have implications. It is therefore a kind of symbolic narrative – a story with roots and branches. It is not simply a pleasant event in a life – it is an experience with the potential to lead on to other things. And in this inheres its subjective significance to a life. However, the fascinating and distinguishing aspect of scientific creativity is the further constraint that the *content* of scientific PEs should be 'objectively' valid and accepted by the community of co-scientists. Scientific knowledge must not merely be compelling to the scientist who thought of it, but should also fit with the best of current information and have the potential for future testability, peer group consensus and reliability in practice.

Limitations of the peak experience

It is perhaps tempting to assume that the peak experience is some kind of guarantee of the truth of a scientific insight. However, this cannot be the case – science is not under-written by a subjective sense of conviction, but rather it should be usable by anyone competent. Delusions are all too common, and people can believe *almost* any proposition with absolute, unshakable confidence. Furthermore, nearly all scientific insights, however valuable in the short term, will turn out to be mistaken or only approximate in the longer term. Yet the peak experience is not wholly irrelevant to the concept of truth at the individual level.

Peak experiences may be associated with insights that are wrong but for the right reasons. In other words, the scientist has done the best possible job of making sense of things at that particular stage in history, but later developments will overthrow their insight. Indeed, this is the usual fate of scientific knowledge. Equally, PEs may also be associated with insights that are right, but for the wrong reasons – the scientist happens to have hit upon the right answer, but used a non-valid method of getting there. Some of the early astronomers, such as Kepler, were number mystics, which led them to seek new planets in order to make them reach a magical figure of seven. They found the extra planet they sought, but were wrong about why it was there – as became apparent when even more planets turned up to spoil the mystic symmetry.

On the other hand, there are scientific peak experiences where – despite a strong and subjectively profound sense of personal conviction – the scientist is wrong and for the wrong reasons. Mathematicians, in particular, are prone to assume that their peak experience-inducing insights, which may be valid in the axiomatic world of mathematics, will inevitably be reflected in the real world where their assumptions have not been confirmed. This kind of thinking is currently widespread in the speculations of 'chaos' and 'complexity' theorists in theoretical biology, as well as in the field of consciousness studies. You can't get peanuts out of oranges, as my old chemistry teacher used to say, and likewise you cannot get biology out of mathematics – the relevant knowledge of causes and entities must be present before crystallisation can occur.

The meaning of the peak experience

If peak experiences are not a guarantee of objective truth, what do they signify? My hunch is that a scientific peak experience is some kind of personal guarantee of the subjective truth of an insight. In other words, scientific peak experiences are a marker which the mind attaches to those of its insights which the mind considers most profound – albeit having made that decision largely as a result of unconscious, inaccessible processing. The peak experience is therefore a signal that states 'This is good stuff, by your standards – maybe the best you are capable of, under current circumstances. Don't ignore it, don't forget it, and try to understand it.'

The peak experience seems to function as a means of focusing attention. The characteristic emotion asserts that the marked insight is something we should dwell upon, puzzle over, sort out – *do* something about. It seems to me that a vital component of the peak experience is exactly this sense of a call to action in the sense of making a decision, changing our lives. It is not – or should not be – simply a passive feeling of happiness and insight. Indeed, episodes of quiescent bliss and idiosyncratically personal insight are easily confused with peak experiences.

The crucial variables relate to knowledge base and brain state. A peak experience cannot generate valid new theories unless the person has sufficient knowledge of the field. There has to be something dissolved in the solution before crystallisation can occur. There are an infinite number of wrong theories, and only a few right ones. There is a negligible probability that the right ones will crystallise out unless the right ingredients are *somewhere* in the solution.

Delirious delights

Cerebral pathology, intoxication with pharmaceutical agents, the clouding of consciousness on the borders of sleep, or the reduced consciousness of sleep itself are all associated with the production of pseudo-peak experiences. Any peak experience that occurs when the brain is functionally impaired (i.e. delirious) is automatically suspect.

Clouding may induce strange outcomes. William James described the effects of alcohol in promoting the 'mystical' faculty, and documented the 'transcendental' experiences of people under the influence of anaesthetic agents such as nitrous oxide (laughing gas) and chloroform. Such agents were able to elicit the sense of direct access to God and led to an embryonic anaesthetic-based 'psychedelic' religious cult during the nineteenth century. More recently, during the 1960s, there were similar claims made for special insights being obtained as a result of the use of 'mind-expanding' hallucinogens such as LSD, mescaline or peyote. Contemporary 'New Age' pharmacological mystics advocate the drug 'Ecstasy' (MDMA) combined with prolonged dancing to pulsating electronic music and flashing lights.

These pharmacological manoeuvres are supposed to provide peak experiences 'on tap', but all of them in fact produce brain impairment. Critical faculties are lowered and euphoric states induced, so that mundane insights take on apparently profound importance. However, only those who are equally 'stoned' find the results impressive.

Another argument made in favour of the benefits of inducing peak experiences is that intoxication removes sensory barriers and experiential filters – allegedly put in place by a repressive social system – to enable a greater immediacy of perception. According to this view, knowledge is 'out there' ready formed and awaiting the apprehending mind. Drugs presumably are believed to render the mind permeable, so as to 'blot up' the truth.

Such notions assume that people are naturally and spontaneously 'creative', but have creativity crushed out of them by societal controls, maladaptive learning, capitalism and other nasty things. This kind of analysis leads to advocating the use of consciousness-altering drugs as a self-educational tool – a technique to 'open the doors of perception' and unbottle spontaneous genius. Intoxication is assumed to remove sensory barriers and experiential filters, break up rigid patterns of unnatural thinking and allow the melted mind to recrystallise in conformity with underlying truth. Aldous Huxley expressed this view in perhaps its most extreme form when he suggested that the human mind knew everything in the universe, but had evolved a filtering mechanism (a 'valve') in order to avoid becoming overwhelmed with stimuli. The peak experience (induced in his case by mescaline) had the effect of releasing this perceptual valve and allowing more of reality to get through to awareness, giving access to otherwise arcane knowledge concerning events and entities in the universe of which we have no direct experience.

Creativity is here seen as something to be liberated. It is sometimes claimed that by rendering apparently peak experiences more common and controllable, drugs may allow the attainment of a 'higher' form of human evolution.

Sorry to be boring, but...

Evolutionary theory takes exactly the opposite view to Huxley. Instead of humans 'naturally' knowing everything and evolving the ability to experience less, biology sees the starting point in insentient, inert matter and regards the capacity to perceive anything at all as having evolved gradually over many millions of years.

Knowledge is certainly *not* out there waiting to burst in on our minds as soon as intoxication lets it through. Rather, the capacity to acquire knowledge, to perceive and to be aware of our perceptions are all adaptations that have been painstakingly constructed over an evolutionary time scale. Moreover, scientific creativity is not spontaneous, natural or preformed, but rather it is attained by constructive human striving – something made, not a spontaneous fact of nature.

No scientific breakthroughs have ever come from ignorant and uneducated prodigies who happened to be intoxicated, nor does creativity in science emerge like a beautiful butterfly breaking free from a chrysalis of social convention. Rather, such creativity is something constructed by efforts and gifts (and luck), including the efforts and gifts of colleagues. Science requires knowledge and skill as well as the right state of mind.

Consciousness as a story-teller

Human consciousness operates as a story-telling device. The somatic marker mechanism associates perceptions with emotions in working memory, so that thought is accompanied by a flow of emotions. These emotions in turn generate a flow of expectations or predictions, which the story may either confirm, or else may contradict in interesting ways that can retrospectively be seen to flow from what went before by less obvious paths, and thus may not be contradictory after all. What makes a story is essentially this flow of linked emotions, a bodily enactment of physical states that have been associated with those propositions which we use in internal modelling.

Consciousness always seems to ascribe causality – it is not content with recording detached representations, but works by synthesising events into a linked linear stream which is then projected into the future as a predictive model to guide behaviour. As bodily emotions fluctuate, feedback to the brain will monitor and interpret this flux in terms of the meaning of perceptions – the emotions interpret the perceptions. As the somatic marker mechanism is a device for using emotions to infer intentions and other states of mind, then sequences of emotions will automatically create inferred narratives of quasi-social relationships – in other words, stories.

Consciousness is so compulsive a story-teller as to be a master confabulator – it will always invent a story in terms of cause-and-effect relations, even when it has no idea what is going on, and the available data are inadequate or contradictory. Young children will interpret abstract computer images that 'pursue' and 'flee' and 'hit' one another in terms of exactly these social behaviours – they will give the abstract shapes personalities and intentions even though they are merely shapes moving on a screen. Seeing faces in the fire, or animals in the clouds, is another instance of the same kind of nearly automatic meaning-generation.

Theoretical science works largely by analogy – by modelling. Perhaps no one can reason in utter abstraction. Scientists build simplified working models of reality, and map these models on to reality to make predictions, seeking a one-to-one correspondence between the model and the world. Some scientific models are mathematical, where real-world entities are mapped on to mathematical symbols and real-world causes are summarised in mathematical operations – such as Einstein's theory of special relativity, $e = mc^2$, where e stands for energy, m stands for mass and c is a very large number. Mathematical predictions can then be tested against observation to see whether the model corresponds to reality.

Other models are much simpler – the 'ball-and-spring' models to show atoms and chemical bonds and valencies, and a host of idiosyncratic mental models which are used to make breakthroughs and are then discarded, often unacknowledged. The molecular shapes used by Crick and Watson to construct their model of the double helix of DNA are a well-known example. The models represented the shape of molecules and some of their ways of bonding to each other, and physically manipulating the shapes was a vital element in solving the structure of DNA. Indeed the 'eureka moment' probably occurred when Watson put together cardboard shapes of the bases and saw that they formed specific complementary pairings. The great physicist Clark Maxwell's notebook musings about how electromagnetism works strike modern observers as extraordinarily 'childish', with their peculiar shapes and swirls representing how magnetism and electricity might operate – yet they none the less led this first-rate genius to the insights that enabled several major breakthroughs in theoretical physics.

The social nature of scientific models

Stories are perhaps the commonest mode of analogical thought. The link between story-telling and scientific theorising is instructive. A scientific hypothesis is like a story in the sense that entities and causal processes are analogous to characters and their motivations. I would guess that – at a deep level – the science and the story-telling processes of the conscious mind are identical; it is the ingredients that differ. It has even been suggested that theoretical physicists and chemists endow their musings with human-like qualities, just as chess masters constantly deploy 'battle' metaphors to describe their strategies in what would otherwise appear to be the most objective and mathematical of games.

Certainly I find that I develop emotions about all aspects of science. For example, I must admit to an idiotic prefer-ence for adrenergic over cholinergic neurotransmitters, because the adrenergic system was associated with physical action (e.g. the 'adrenalin rush'), while cholinergic activity had connotations of lying around feeling bloated after a meal (acetylcholinergic fibres innervate the gut). Silly, of course, but I couldn't help anthropomorphising about entities which were important to me.

I would go so far as to suggest that creative science is *constrained anthropomorphism*. Learning to do a science involves learning how to tell a particular kind of story – who the important characters are and what are their typical causal motivations – that is the anthropomorphism. Each scientific discipline has a distinctive set of personalities and behaviours. In physics, there might be fundamental particles acted on by gravitational, electromagnetic and nuclear forces. In biology, there might be cells and organ-isms acted on by macromolecules such as DNA and proteins under the influence of natural selection.

The constraint comes in because the range of possible stories that one is permitted to tell about particular entities is strictly limited by previous relevant science. Thus whether the entities in the story are attracted or repelled, counterbalanced or exaggerated, additive or multiplicative in their effects, these aspects are controlled strictly by scientific criteria.

However, having established a proper set of 'dispositions, motivations and intentions' for the entities, we predict what they will do by exactly the kind of 'story-generating' social intelligence that we have been exploring in the earlier parts of this book. Indeed, I would go so far as to say that most people can *only* be creative in this quasi-narrative fashion, and scientific creativity involves story-telling of a highly specialised kind. The exception is mathematics, where the outcome of interacting entities is determined not by quasi-social factors but by mathematical functions.

The role of narrative is both to generate theories and to make them usable – because science is a human product, it needs to be shaped to the human mind. If a scientific theory cannot be put into a quasi-social shape, then we find it very difficult to think about. Our mind, after all, is bubbling with social meaning even when the world is chaotic – we see pictures in random dots, and monsters in the shadows. We confabulate causal pathways to explain our emotions and behaviours. Inanimate objects such as stones, rivers and trees are imbued with personality and powers of malevolence or benignity. For humans, the world is full of relevance and purpose. Reality comes to us already imprinted with labels of preference. Theories that cannot be subsumed to this world do not have much chance of being remembered or used, as they will be forced aside by more 'interesting' ideas.

Thus it is a fusion of constrained reality, trained aesthetic appreciation and emotional preference that makes possible the scientific peak experience. The peak experience is that moment when analogy strikes us – we see underlying unity, similarity in difference, meaning emerging from chaos, a bunch of disconnected facts coalescing into a story.

Conclusion

Peak experiences are an accidental by-product of human social intelligence and we are constrained to view the world through spectacles of social intelligence. This applies to science as well as the arts – both endeavours are intensely subjective, and the difference lies in the social validity of their insights rather than the mode of generation.

The significance of a peak experience is essentially subjective. The apparently self-validating emotion of deep and profound significance which sweeps like a wave across clear consciousness is probably a somatic marker informing us that we have performed cognitions of special importance and significance to our own goals, and rewarding us with ecstatic feelings for having done so. It is analogous to the satisfaction of a good story well told – a story with the ring of truth to it.

The subjective importance of the peak experience is considerable. It has a talismanic function – something remembered as a reward for difficult but desirable behaviour in the immediate past, something pointing towards a fruitful line of behaviour for the longer-term future.

The objective validity of the scientific peak experience is determined by its public dimension – that is, whether it stands up to testing by peers. However, the predictive value to be placed upon a hypothesis arrived at during a peak experience is not wholly arbitrary. It is a product of the quality of the scientist. In the first place, a scientist must be *competent* to assert the hypothesis – they should have a mind that is informed and unclouded. The *probable* objective validity of a scientific peak experience is affected by the quality of the scientist's thinking and preparation, and how well they have internalised the processes and constraints of their discipline.

Peak experience insights have the potential to mislead as well as to enlighten. The easy induction of pseudo-profound insights by intoxicants serves as a warning of the potential pitfalls. When the mind is deranged by drugs, delirium or drowsiness, then this emotion may short-circuit and 'spontaneously discharge' to become attached to almost any event – such as an idiosyncratic pronunciation of the word '*Coll-oh-nell*' or the importance of an exclamation mark. Then an arbitrary object or stimulus becomes labelled with an obscure sense of delight and personal relevance. When the brain is impaired, the specific object to which the sense of significance attaches itself may be a matter of chance, and the insights may be nonsensical – a process we might call the *Colonel Flastratus phenomenon*, where portentous meaning is projected on to an irrelevant stimulus. By making the peak experience easier, and by severing affect from cognition, intoxication also diminishes its meaningfulness.

Peak experiences are the result of a 'significance alarm' going off in the brain. When things are working properly, this alarm will only be triggered when something 'important' has happened that is worthy of sustained attention. Thus we are often right to take peak experiences seriously – yet their 'significance' is seldom transparent, and we cannot take the insights of peak experiences at face value. Perhaps the best approach is to regard them as a fascinating enigma – a code which may contain a message of profound import.

On the other hand, after laboriously cracking the cipher, we may not find the secret of life at all, but merely a pointless pun.

Further reading and references

Chapter 1 – Psychiatry and the human condition

The background to this chapter, and to the book as a whole, arises from a conference I attended at University College London on 4–5 March 1998, which was organised by Carl Elliott. I prepared a talk for this conference which was later published in the *Journal of the Royal Society of Medicine* as 'Psychopharmacology and the human condition', and had formative discussions with David Healy and Peter Kramer, who were also participants. The general idea of psychiatric illness as a common fact of everyday life had previously been provoked by Healy's *The Suspended Revolution* and *The Antidepressant Era,* and Kramer's *Listening to Prozac*. In particular, I was stimulated by grappling with the implications of the fact that 'antidepressants' often benefited people who did not fulfil the criteria of major depressive disorder.

Since 1994 I have been involved in the emerging field of evolutionary psychology, and have been interested by recent progress in evolutionary biology, especially as it applies to humans and human behaviour. My interest was first caught by Matt Ridley's *The Red Queen*, which concentrated mainly on sexual selection, and then by the trailblazing edited volume *The Adapted Mind*. In a chapter of *The Adapted Mind*, and in *Darwin, Sex and Status*, the anthropologist Jerome F Barkow showed how an evolutionary perspective could throw light on human culture. More of this approach came from Jared Diamond in *The Rise and Fall of the Third Chimpanzee*, which drew my attention to the egalitarian and leisured society of our nomadic foraging ancestors, the transition to agriculture, and the major idea of James Woodburn's that societies could be divided into 'immediate-return and delayed-return' economies (which constitutes one of the most valid and profound categories in the social sciences, in my view). The work of Ernest Gellner on types of human society and the transitions between them confirmed and sharpened these insights.

My description of ancestral human culture is, of course, a matter of probability rather than absolute certainty. The major features are highly likely to be correct, but details would surely have varied between times and places.

References

Barkow JH (1989) *Darwin, Sex and Status*. Toronto: University of Toronto Press.

Gellner E (1988) *Plough, Sword and Book: The Structure of Human History*. London: Collins.

Further reading

Barkow JH, Cosmides L and Tooby J (eds) (1992). *The Adapted Mind*. New York: Oxford University Press.

Bird-David N (1992) Beyond 'the original affluent society': a culturalist reformulation (and replies). *Curr Anthropol*. **33**: 25–47.

Byrne RW and Whiten A (1988) *Machiavellian Intelligence: Social Expertise and the Evolution of Intellect in Monkeys, Apes and Humans*. Oxford: Clarendon Press.

Charlton BG (1997) The inequity of inequality: egalitarian instincts and evolutionary psychology. *J Health Psychol*. **2**: 413–25.

Charlton BG (1998) Psychopharmacology and the human condition. *J R Soc Med*. **91**: 599–601.

Cohen M and Armelagos G (eds) (1984) *Paleopathology at the Origin of Agriculture.* Orlando, FL: Academic Press.

Diamond J (1992) *The Rise and Fall of the Third Chimpanzee.* London: Vintage.

Erdal D and Whiten A (1996) Egalitarianism and Machiavellian intelligence in human evolution. In: PA Mellars and KR Gibson (eds) *Modelling the Early Human Mind.* Cambridge: Cambridge McDonald Institute for Archaeological Research, 139–50.

Healy D (1990) *The Suspended Revolution.* London: Faber.

Kramer PD (1994) *Listening to Prozac.* London: Fourth Estate.

Ridley M (1993). *The Red Queen: Sex and the Evolution of Human Behaviour.* London: Viking.

Sahlins M (1968) Notes on the original affluent society. In: RB Lee and I DeVore (eds) *Man the Hunter.* Chicago: Aldine, 85–9.

Woodburn J (1982) Egalitarian societies. *Man.* 17: 431–51.

Chapter 2 – Social intelligence and the somatic marker mechanism

The profoundly important concept of social intelligence originates with Nicholas Humphrey, and has been taken up and extended in the 'Machiavellian intelligence' volumes by Andrew Whiten and Richard Byrne. This work merges into the literature concerning the concept of 'theory of mind' which I explored particularly in the work of Simon Baron Cohen and his colleagues who were interested in autism. However, I have introduced a distinction between here-and-now tactical social intelligence (common to many animals) and *strategic* social intelligence based on internally modelling and evaluating social interactions (which is probably confined to a few species of social mammals). It is strategic social intelligence that is distinctive although possibly not unique to the primate lineage, and which probably best deserves the 'Machiavellian' sobriquet.

The nature of strategic social intelligence depends on the nature of the mechanism which performs it – that is, the somatic marker mechanism as described in the work of Antonio R Damasio and his colleagues, especially in the book *Descartes' Error*. The idea of the somatic marker mechanism is expounded more fully in Appendix 1. The crucial fact that emerges from Damasio's analysis is that emotions are body states, and that the most obvious way to affect emotion is to affect its bodily expression. As psychiatric illness is often dominated by changes in emotion, this provides a way of understanding psychiatric drug action. Any drug that affects the body will potentially affect emotion, and selectivity of peripheral action is a plausible mechanism whereby drugs might exert *specific* emotional effects.

The usual idea is that psychiatric drugs work on the brain in very specific ways. My general view is that most drugs that really do work on the brain do so by having pretty crude and general effects on overall brain activity, producing crude and general behavioural effects such as sedation or arousal – and that tolerance to these effects develops quite rapidly.

So I shall argue that most psychiatric drugs exert either general effects on the brain leading to general effects on behaviour, or specific effects on the body leading to specific effects on behaviour.

In reality, the concepts outlined here, such as working memory (WM) and the somatic marker mechanism (SMM) are considerably more complex than can be presented in these schematic notes.

For instance, Damasio highlights the way in which the SMM, as it exists in humans, can bypass the body itself and use 'as-if' mechanisms. These 'as-if' processes probably operate on somatic representations from the brainstem on up to the cortex. Emotions are largely body states, but brain states also contribute. This implies that the SMM may still be used in conditions in which a somatic marker is created inside the brain itself.

Working memory is not really a place or a site, but a process. And the WM process is situated in several places, including the prefrontal cortex but also (for example) in primary and secondary sensory cortices. The point is that integration between cognitive representations occurs on-line, and depends on the 'holding' function of working memory. Finally, it is worth emphasising that somatic marking can occur non-consciously, as well as consciously.

References for this area are provided in the section below on Appendix 1.

Chapter 3 – Psychiatric classification

My interest in psychiatric classification goes back to my time as a medical student and in clinical practice during the early 1980s. Harrison Pope drew my attention to the fact that diagnostic categories could be misleading as a guide to prognosis and treatment unless account was also taken of the prominent symptoms. Eric Wood told me of the US studies in which psychotic patients randomised to imipramine and chlorpromazine were found to respond by symptoms rather than by diagnosis, and I became sympathetic to Tim Crow's then concept of a 'unitary psychosis'. I learned a great deal of neuroendocrinology science from the likes of Nicol Ferrier, Phil Lowry and Alan Leake. I was also aware that the action of psychiatric drugs did not conform to such categories as 'antidepressant' or 'neuroleptic', and that we needed a different – and probably symptom-based – way of understanding these questions.

By 1990 I was persuaded that the existing strategies of psychiatric research were going nowhere, and I argued this in a somewhat notorious paper that was published in *Psychological Medicine*. However, I had little idea of what to do instead, except to adapt the approach of cognitive neuropsychology which I read about in Tim Shallice's book *From Neuropsychology to Mental Structure*, and in works by John Marshall, and which I discussed with my friend Janice Kay who was working on aphasia. In 1992 I read David Healy's *The Suspended Revolution*, which persuaded me of the need for a more 'phenomenological' kind of psychiatry, with attention paid to reports of subjective psychological states. Shortly afterwards, Tony David published an exciting editorial in *Psychological Medicine* about the proposed field of cognitive neuropsychiatry. However, as I had no new ideas about clinical practice, therapy or drug development, these criticisms were rendered pretty narrowly 'academic' and a matter only for pure research.

The breakthrough in understanding psychiatric drugs was also made through reading David Healy's publications – specifically the series of books comprising *Psychiatric Drugs Explained*, *The Psychopharmacologists* (Volumes I and II), and *The Antidepressant Era* – but also by conversations and correspondence with the man himself.

When Healy's phenomenology and psychopharmacological insights were combined with cognitive neuropsychiatry, cognitive neuroscience (of which I had become aware since joining the Department of Psychology at Newcastle) and my own basis of evolutionary biology, at long last a new way of looking at mental illness and its treatment began to crystallise. I saw that the task of a new and biologically valid approach to clinical psychiatry was to describe and classify categories of 'psychiatric' symptoms and to 'match' this nosology with categories of drug effects. Each patient's condition could then be treated in an individually tailored fashion, and the clinician (or the patient him- or herself) would know what aspect of the illness the drug was trying to treat – which would potentially enable the minimum effective dose to be established, again on an individual basis. Damasio's theory of emotions alerted me to look at the body rather than the brain as a basis for the emotional states characteristic of psychiatric illness. The final step was to return to clinical work, attending ward rounds and speaking to patients, and to seek to confirm these ideas by observing patients' experience of symptoms and responses to drugs. This triggered more ideas. Then it was a matter of writing it all down, which takes us up to the present...

Further reading

Caramazza A (1986) On drawing inferences about the structure of normal cognitive systems from the analysis of patterns of impaired performance: the cases for single patient studies. *Brain Cogn.* **5**: 41–66.

Charlton BG (1990) A critique of biological psychiatry. *Psychol Med.* **20**: 3–6.

Charlton BG and Walston F (1998) Individual case studies in clinical research. *J Eval Clin Pract.* **4**: 147–55.

Damasio AR (1994) *Descartes' Error: Emotion, Reason and the Human Brain.* New York: Putnam.

David A (1993) Cognitive neuropsychiatry? *Psychol Med.* **23**: 1–5.

Healy D (1992) *The Suspended Revolution.* London: Faber.

Healy D (1996) *The Psychopharmacologists.* London: Altman.

Healy D (1997) *Psychiatric Drugs Explained.* London: Mosby.

Healy D (1998) *The Psychopharmacologists II.* London: Altman.

Healy D (1998) *The Antidepressant Era.* Cambridge, MA: Harvard University Press.

Marshall JC and Newcombe F (1984) Putative problems and pure progress in neuropsychological single-case studies. *J Clin Neuropsychol.* **6**: 65–70.

Shallice T (1988) *From Neuropsychology to Mental Structure.* Cambridge: Cambridge University Press.

Chapter 4 – The delusional disorders *and* Chapter 5 – Bizarre delusions

The original idea for these chapters also came from some comments about the ordinary, everyday nature of paranoia by David Healy in *The Suspended Revolution*. This insight preyed on my mind for several years, until I saw a way to combine it with an evolutionary perspective and the implications of the somatic marker mechanism. The whole approach was refined during a year-long and extremely detailed phenomenological case study of persecutory delusions I undertook with Florence Walston, who was at that time a medical student. In conversations with Hamish McClelland we were able to draw on his unparalleled clinical experience to confirm and refine these ideas.

Thus we developed the hypothesis of 'theory-of-mind' delusions.

The category of *bizarre* delusions emerged as a consequence of the need to differentiate the truly 'mad' ideas of brain-impaired people from false beliefs that emerge logically from 'mistaken' inferences about what other people are thinking or intending. Although consistent with what I have gleaned of clinical experience and from the literature, the section on bizarre delusions is primarily speculative and theoretical. I hope that someone will soon take the opportunity to test this formally.

Further reading

Baron-Cohen S (1990) Autism: a specific cognitive disorder of 'mind-blindness'. *Int Rev Psychiatry.* 2: 81–90.

Brothers L (1990) The social brain: a project for integrating primate behavior and neurophysiology in a new domain. *Concepts Neurosci.* 1: 27–51.

Buss DM (1994) *The Evolution of Desire.* New York: Basic Books.

Byrne RW and Whiten A (eds) (1988) *Machiavellian Intelligence: Social Expertise and the Evolution of Intellect in Monkeys, Apes and Humans.* Oxford: Clarendon Press.

Charlton BG (in press) Theory of mind and the 'somatic marker mechanism' (SMM). *Behav Brain Sci.*

Charlton BG and McClelland HA (1999) Theory of mind and the delusional disorders. *J Nerv Ment Dis.* 187: 380–3.

Charlton BG and Walston F (1998) Individual case studies in clinical research. *J Eval Clin Pract.* 4: 147–55.

Damasio AR (1994) *Descartes' Error: Emotion, Reason and the Human Brain.* New York: Putnam.

Dunbar R (1996) *Grooming, Gossip and the Evolution of Language.* London: Faber.

Garety PA and Hemsley DR (1994) *Delusions: Investigations into the Psychology of Delusional Reasoning.* Hove: Psychology Press.

Geary DC, Rumsey M, Bow-Thomas CC and Hoard MK (1995) Sexual jealousy as a facultative trait: evidence from the pattern of sex differences in adults from China and the United States. *Ethol Sociobiol.* **16**: 355–83.

Walston F, David AS and Charlton BG (1998) Sex differences in the content of persecutory delusions: a reflection of hostile threats in the ancestral environment? *Evol Hum Behav.* **19**: 257–60.

Whiten A and Byrne RW (eds) (1997) *Machiavellian Intelligence II: Extensions and Evaluations.* Cambridge: Cambridge University Press.

Wiederman MW and Allgeier ER (1993) Gender differences in sexual jealousy: adaptionist or social learning explanation? *Ethol Sociobiol.* **14**: 115–40.

Wilson M and Daly M (1992) The man who mistook his wife for a chattel. In: JH Barkow, L Cosmides and J Tooby (eds) *The Adapted Mind: Evolutionary Psychology and the Generation of Culture.* New York: Oxford University Press, 289–322.

Chapter 6 – Delirium and brain impairment

The absence of delirium in patients diagnosed as suffering from one of the 'functional psychoses' (syndromes such as schizophrenia, mania and depression) lies at the very heart of the neo-Kraepelinian nosology. My heretical idea that is that – contrary to this doctrine – patients with functional psychoses who have symptoms of hallucinations, bizarre delusions and thought disorder *must* instead be functionally brain impaired and therefore suffering from delirium. This view (which will strike many clinicians as absurd or foolish) was more or less forced upon me by trying to understand the cognitive mechanisms behind (in particular) auditory hallucinations in the context of contemporary knowledge about how the brain works.

Paul Janssen's interview with David Healy in *The Psychopharmacologists* (Volume II) was a revelation of the significance of sleep to normal human functioning, and the importance of chronic, severe sleep deprivation in many psychiatric syndromes – in particular the following sentence: 'What always struck me was that so many chronic schizophrenics not only hallucinate and have delusions and difficulty to establish human contact, but they also complain of sleep disturbances and if we actually objectively measure their EEG it is very abnormal'. Janssen also pointed out the effectiveness of risperidone in producing increased deep sleep (as measured on EEG). The obvious implication (not explicitly made by Janssen) is that it is sleep disturbance which causes the hallucinations and delusions (rather than the reverse), that the 'abnormal' EEG is evidence of delirium in these patients (an abnormal EEG implies abnormal brain function) and that the 'antipsychotic' effect is at least partly produced by the effect of increasing deep sleep.

My own clinical enquiries into the history of the psychiatric patients I was seeing confirmed that true psychotic phenomena always seemed to be accompanied by either severe sleep deprivation or some other cause of delirium (e.g. drug intoxication), that the mental state of these patients could plausibly be interpreted as a light state of delirium, and that clinical improvement was often preceded by an improvement in sleep. The most obvious conclusion is that chronic severe sleep deprivation causes the delirium, the delirium causes the psychotic symptoms, and induction of sleep by 'tranquillising' drugs is what alleviates psychotic symptoms. Unfortunately, I have not been able to perform the EEG research studies which might confirm or refute this, but the idea appears to be compatible with the literature on EEG in psychotic illnesses, including some excellent but largely forgotten work from the 1950s and 1960s.

Further reading

Charlton BG (1995) Psychiatric implications of surgery and critical care. In: MA Glasby and CL-H Huang (eds) *Applied Physiology for Surgery and Critical Care*. London: Butterworth-Heinemann, 739–42.

Janssen P (1998) From haloperidol to risperidone. In: D Healy (ed.) *The Psychopharmacologists II*. London: Altman, 39–70.

Lipowski ZJ (1990) *Delirium: Acute Confusional States.* New York: Oxford University Press.

Niedermeyer E and da Silva L (1993) *Electroencephalography: Basic Principles, Clinical Applications and Related Fields.* Baltimore, MD: Williams and Williams.

Sims A (1995) *Symptoms in the Mind.* London: WB Saunders.

Slater E and Roth M (1977) *Clinical Psychiatry* (3e). London: Balliere Tindall.

Stromgren LS (1997) ECT in acute delirium and related clinical states. *Convuls Ther.* **13**: 10–17.

Wehr TA (1990) Effects of wakefulness and sleep on depression and mania. In: J Montplaisir and R Godbout (eds) *Sleep and Biological Rhythms: Basic Mechanisms and Applications.* New York: Oxford University Press, 42–86.

Chapter 7 – The 'anti-delirium' theory of electroconvulsive therapy (ECT) action

Having made the link between chronic, severe sleep deprivation and the kind of psychotic phenomena that are seen in the most severe instances of depression, then the probable nature of ECT action became much clearer. The idea that ECT might work primarily in those depressed patients who were delirious (by the definitions of the previous chapter, and usually as a consequence of sleep deprivation) seems to fit with early research into ECT action, and also explains why ECT often benefits patients with acute mania (which many people consider to be the 'opposite' of depression). This was strikingly confirmed by observing the immediate resolution of chronic, intractable, non-neuroleptic responsive mania following a single ECT treatment and sound sleep.

Since this book went to press, I have discovered the work of J Lee Kavanan – which I believe constitutes a convincing explanation for the 'anti-delirium' effects of ECT. I have added two references to this author's remarkable body of theoretical work.

Further reading

Abrams R (1997) *Electroconvulsive Therapy* (3e). New York: Oxford University Press.

Carney MWP, Roth M and Garside RF (1965) The diagnosis of depressive symptoms and the prediction of ECT response. *Br J Psychiatry*. **111**: 659–74.

Charlton BG (1995) Psychiatric implications of surgery and critical care. In: MA Glasby and CL-H Huang (eds) *Applied Physiology for Surgery and Critical Care*. London: Butterworth-Heinemann, 739–42.

Charlton BG (1999) The 'anti-delirium' theory of electroconvulsive therapy action. *Med Hypotheses*. **52**: 609–11.

Fink M and Sackeim S (1996) Convulsive therapy in schizophrenia? *Schizophr Bull*. **22**: 27–39.

Kavanan JL (1997) Memory, sleep and the evolution of mechanisms of synaptic efficiency maintenance. *Neurosci*. **79**: 7–44.

Kavanan JL (1999) Adaptations and pathologies linked to dynamic stabilization of neural circuitry. *Neurosci Biobehav Rev*. **23**: 635–48.

Lipowski ZJ (1990) *Delirium: Acute Confusional States*. New York: Oxford University Press.

Niedermeyer E and da Silva L (1993) *Electroencephalography: Basic Principles, Clinical Applications, and Related Fields*. Baltimore, MD: Williams and Williams.

Slater E and Roth M (1977) *Clinical Psychiatry* (3e). London: Balliere Tindall.

Small JG, Klapper MH, Kellams JJ, Miller MJ, Milstein V, Sharpley PH and Small IF (1988) ECT compared with lithium in the management of manic states. *Arch Gen Psychiatry*. **45**: 727–32.

Stromgren LS (1997) ECT in acute delirium and related clinical states. *Convuls Ther*. **13**: 10–17.

Wehr TA (1990) Effects of wakefulness and sleep on depression and mania. In: J Montplaisir and R Godbout (eds) *Sleep and Biological Rhythms: Basic Mechanisms and Applications*. New York: Oxford University Press, 42–86.

Chapter 8 – The malaise theory of depression

For me, this is the most exciting idea in the book, since it is the culmination of nearly two decades of (albeit intermittent) intensive research, reading and thinking about the nature of depression. Given this, perhaps I may be forgiven the *hubris* of suggesting that this theoretical framework offers considerable potential for improving the lives of large numbers of people, although naturally this cannot be known for sure unless or until formal studies to test the ideas begin to emerge.

Once again the germ of the idea comes from a remark of David Healy's in *The Suspended Revolution*, which stuck in my mind. The penny finally dropped during a ward round when I asked a 'depressed' in-patient AK whether she felt *ill* – and she turned to look hard at me and said vehemently 'Yes! And that is the first time anyone has asked me that.' This insight was further explored in a series of in-depth phenomenological interviews for which I am extremely grateful to AK. The immunological side of this theory was very usefully checked over by presenting a paper to the immunologists' club at Newcastle General Hospital, and by the convenor of that club, Consultant Clinical Immunologist Dr Gavin Spickett.

Further reading

Charlton BG (1998) Psychopharmacology and the human condition. *J R Soc Med*. **91**: 599–601.

Charlton BG (2000) The malaise theory of depression: major depressive disorder is sickness behaviour and antidepressants are analgesic. *Med Hypotheses*. **54**: 126–30.

Connor TJ and Leonard BE (1998) Depression, stress and immunological activation: the role of cytokines in depressive disorders. *Life Sci*. **62**: 583–606.

Damasio AR (1994) *Descartes' Error: Emotion, Reason and the Human Brain*. New York: Putnam.

Hart BL (1988) Biological basis of the behavior of sick animals. *Neurosci Biobehav Rev.* **12**: 123–37.

Healy D (1990) *The Suspended Revolution.* London: Faber.

Healy D (1996) *Psychiatric Drugs Explained.* London: Mosby-Wolfe.

Hickie I and Lloyd A (1995) Are cytokines associated with neuropsychiatric syndromes in humans? *Int J Immunopharmacol.* **17**: 677–83.

Joyce PR, Hawes CR, Mulder RT, Sellman JD, Wilson DA and Boswell DR (1992) Elevated levels of acute-phase plasma proteins in depression. *Biol Psychiatry.* **32**: 1035–41.

Kent S, Bluthe R-M, Kelley KW and Dantzer R (1992) Sickness behavior as a new target for drug development. *Trends Pharmacol Sci.* **12**: 24–8.

Maes M (1993) A review on the acute-phase response in major depression. *Rev Neurosci.* **4**: 407–16.

Maes M, Bosmans E, Suy E, Vandervost C, Dejonckheere C, Minner B and Raus J (1991) Depression-related disturbances in mitogen-induced lymphocyte responses, interleukin 1-beta, and soluble interleukin-2-receptor production. *Acta Psychiatr Scand.* **84**: 379–86.

Maier SF and Watkins LR (1999) Bidirectional communication between the brain and the immune system: implications for behavior. *Animal Behav.* **57**: 741–51.

Schneider K (1959) (translated by MW Hamilton and EW Anderson). *Clinical Psychopathology.* New York: Grune and Stratton.

Sims A (1995) *Symptoms in the Mind* (2e). London: WB Saunders.

Smith A, Tyrrell D, Coyle K and Higgins P (1988) Effects of interferon alpha on performance in man. *Psychopharmacology.* **96**: 414–16.

Yirmiya R (1997) Behavioral and psychological effects of immune activation: implications for 'depression due to a general medical condition'. *Curr Opin Psychiatry.* **10**: 470–76.

Chapter 9 – Antidepressant drug action

There is, it turns out, a tremendous amount of supportive evidence in the literature for the idea that depression is sickness behaviour, so the nature of major depressive disorder seemed reasonably clear once that link had been made. However, the mode of action of 'antidepressants' remained obscure until I realised that the link between major depressive disorder and influenza implied that an effective antidepressant would need to be an analgesic or painkiller of the same general type that provides symptomatic relief in influenza.

I already knew that tricyclic 'antidepressants' were used in pain clinics, but had not realised that their analgesic properties were so well established, nor that they were so widely used in the symptomatic and palliative care of cancer and other malaise-related conditions. The complementary implication is that analgesics – especially opiates – should have clinically valuable 'antidepressant' (i.e. anti-malaise) properties, and this view is massively (although inconsistently) supported in the psychiatric literature going back more than a 100 years.

I am still unsure how selective serotonin reuptake inhibitors (SSRIs) fit into this scheme. They certainly differ from tricyclics in their primary mode of therapeutic action, and I am convinced that they are very valuable drugs for some people, and have transformed lives for the better. Direct enquiry from patients and a detailed reading of the literature have led to the idea that the special action may be one of 'emotion-buffering', probably through some kind of stabilising effect on the autonomic nervous system. Certainly SSRIs are more effective in the population of anxiously miserable out-patients than in the populations of 'melancholic, psychotic' in-patients, their analgesic activity is not striking (with the possible exception of fluoxetine) and evidence of their benefits to people with labile emotions (including post-stroke patients) seems to be accumulating. The nature of emotion-buffering requires further exploration, and would seem to be a potentially fruitful area for research.

Further reading

Charlton BG (2000) The malaise theory of depression: major depressive disorder is sickness behaviour and antidepressants are analgesic. *Med Hypotheses.* **54**: 126–30.

Healy D (1997) *Psychiatric Drugs Explained*. London: Mosby.

Healy D (1998) *The Antidepressant Era*. Cambridge, MA: Harvard University Press.

Holland JC, Romano SJ, Heiligenstein JH, Tepner RG and Wilson MG (1998) A controlled trial of fluoxetine and desipramine in depressed women with advanced cancer. *Psychooncology*. 7: 291–300.

Lee R and Spencer PSJ (1977) Antidepressants and pain: a review of the pharmacological data supporting the use of certain tricyclics in chronic pain. *J Int Med Res*. 5 (Supplement 1): 146–56.

McDaniel JS, Musselman DL, Porter MR, Reed DA and Nemeroff CB (1995) Depression in patients with cancer: diagnosis, biology and treatment. *Arch Gen Psychiatry*. 52: 89–99.

Muller H and Moller HJ (1998) Methodological problems in the estimation of the onset of the antidepressant effect. *J Affect Disord*. 48: 15–23.

Panerai AE, Bianchi M, Sacerdote P, Ripamonti C, Ventafridda V and De Conno F (1991) Antidepressants in cancer pain. *J Palliat Care*. 7: 42–4.

Portnoy RK and Kanner RM (1996) *Pain Management: Theory and Practice*. Philadelphia, PA: FA Davis.

Vereby K (ed.) (1982) *Opioids in Mental Illness: Theories, Clinical Observations and Treatment Possibilities*. New York: New York Academy of Science.

Xia Y, DePierre JW and Nassberger L (1996) Tricyclic antidepressants inhibit IL-6, IL-1beta and TNF-alpha release in human blood monocytes and IL-2 and interferon-gamma in T-cells. *Immunopharmacology*. 34: 27–37.

Chapter 10 – Mania

Mania is at the same time one of the most obvious and 'real' of psychiatric illnesses, and one of the hardest to define. In particular, the idea that the manic state should be defined by a 'high' mood has proved to be a red herring. The insight presented here, that the essence of mania is freedom from the negative feedback of fatigue, crystallised from a consideration of the importance of fatigue in depression, and the role of analgesia (such as tricyclics) in removing the symptoms of fatigue. This allowed me to distinguish between a state of 'arousal' and high energy (which is a part of the spectrum of normal life) and the pathological state of 'hypomania' (when this arousal is not limited by the negative feedback of fatigue).

Thus I have come to regard fatigue as being an 'algesic' state, akin to pain – and treatable by painkillers. In other words, fatigue is different from sleepiness. Fatigue is the dysphoric state that leads us to want to rest and to stop activity, whereas sleepiness is the desire for sleep. The two are dissociable, as when one is 'exhausted' with fatigue but cannot sleep. And fatigue can be treated (e.g. with analgesics, such as tricyclics) even when the drug is sedative. So far I have not been able to find anyone else who regards fatigue as an 'algesic state' in quite this manner, although this view certainly seems to be compatible with much of what is known about the subject of fatigue.

If mania was primarily an absence of fatigue, then this implies that chronic amphetamine usage as a pharmacological model of mania might be working less by amphetamine causing arousal (which I had previously assumed was the case), and more by amphetamine causing analgesia. On searching the literature I was astonished to discover that amphetamine is one of the most powerful known analgesics (a fact that has presumably been hushed up because of real but exaggerated fears of amphetamine addiction). Caffeine also turns out to be an analgesic as well as a mild psychostimulant. The whole picture of causes, treatments and consequences fits together in such a neat way that one must take seriously the possibility that it is true!

Rather than providing a set of manufactured references generated *post hoc*, I shall indicate how I went about checking the validity of this theory of mania. In the first place, I already knew – from the seven or so years when I was a full-time neuroendocrinologist and adrenal researcher – quite a lot about endorphins and the other endogenous opiates, and about cortisol and the other glucocorticoids. Predictions about the possible mania-inducing effects of glucocorticoids and opiates were followed up by trawling large swathes through the Medline computerised reference system, and by reading whatever books on this topic were available in the library. My conclusion was that there was a great deal of confirmatory evidence for the proposition that endorphins and glucocorticoids might be anti-fatigue analgesics with a tendency to induce mania, and that the opiate antagonist naloxone probably had an anti-manic effect when given in adequate doses. There were also plenty of published papers that disagreed with this view. However, I felt that these were all sufficiently flawed for me to be able to disregard them. I also read about the physiology of sleep generally, and that seemed to fit, too.

Then there was clinical work. By sheer luck, I was able to see a reasonable number of classic manic patients (perhaps a couple of dozen) through their illness and into recovery, and could check whether or not the natural history of their illnesses was consistent with the natural history predicted by the arousal–analgesia theory. It was. In particular, the idea that chronic severe sleep deprivation is necessary to shift a hypomanic person into full-blown psychotic mania, and that sleep would terminate the psychotic features of mania, seemed to be exactly right. And if the pharmacological treatments were interpreted as hypnotic rather than 'antipsychotic' then the scheme of understanding still worked perfectly.

Therefore I am quite confident about these ideas in relation to mania. Of course, I have been selective about what I believed and disregarded, but not arbitrarily so, as I have an exact and constraining theory against which to test observations. Selectivity in choosing evidence is nothing to be ashamed of – as the greatest living member of my tribe of theoretical biologists (Francis Crick) says in *What Mad Pursuit*, this is just how theoretical science is done. After all, most observational evidence (like most scientific propositions) will turn out to be wrong, so it would be an error to include all of the observational evidence. To generate true theories one *must* discard most of the observational evidence – and if that sounds like a paradox, then think again!

Chapter 11 – Neuroleptics

In current practice, acute mania is treated by sedation and neuroleptics, while 'mood-stabilisers' such as lithium are used to prevent its recurrence when people suffer from frequent repeated episodes of mania (or of mania and depression). Despite their central importance to psychiatry, very little is known at present about the therapeutic action of either neuroleptics or lithium, although a lot is known about their 'side-effects'. (Indeed, there is no information at all in most psychiatric textbooks or even monographs about the clinical therapeutic actions of these drugs. There are sections on supposed molecular-level actions, but nothing whatsoever on psychological or physiological therapeutic effects.) I have come to believe that in the case of both neuroleptics and lithium *the therapeutic action is also one of the main so-called 'side-effects'*.

The action of both neuroleptics and lithium can be described in a general way as blunting of emotions. Damasio's insight is that emotions are actually the brain representations of body states – so that if the *bodily enactment* of emotions is blocked, so will be our experience of these emotions. As neuroleptics (certainly) and lithium (very probably) both block the muscular manifestations of emotion, then this motor action seems an obvious way in which these drugs might produce a blunting of subjective emotion. So although neuroleptics and lithium differ in several respects, it is suggested that they share a primary therapeutic action of impairing the motor manifestations of emotion. This is probably due to an effect on the basal ganglia, with the activity of the latter being impaired such that the muscular enactment of emotions is in turn impaired, and since enactment is impaired so is the subjective perception of emotion. My hunch (and it is just a hunch) is that the nature of motor impairment is different in each case, with neuroleptics producing a kind of 'tonic' impairment, and lithium producing a 'clonic' impairment. This proposition could easily be tested by measuring drug effects during enactment of somatic emotion (such as skin conductance) in response to emotion-inducing stimuli.

Again, I shall refrain from providing an elaborate bibliography. Suffice it to say that a trawl through Medline reveals that there is plenty of literature out there in support of these theories, or at least consistent with them – and little to contradict them. The idea that atypical neuroleptics may be operating primarily as sedative hypnotics comes from Paul Janssen's interview with David Healy in *The Psychopharmacologists II*, and it seems to be consistent with the general run of commentary on 'atypicals' (reading between the lines, sometimes) and my own recent clinical observations. What is needed now is testing in practice, not more literature reviews.

Chapter 12 – Schizophrenia

For the last 20 years I have consistently heard it said by experts that schizophrenia is not one thing but many things. I first heard this idea from Harrison Pope on my student elective to Harvard, and shortly afterwards from Angus Mackay at a journal club in Newcastle, and Tim Crow implied as much with his unitary psychosis ideas. The heterogeneity of schizophrenia (i.e. its lack of biological validity as a unitary category) seems to be mainstream. Nevertheless, the category is continuously used in research and clinical practice, presumably because there is no other available way of conceptualising chronic psychotic patients.

My purpose here is to set out some symptomatic variables which can be used to classify chronic psychotic patients for the purposes of research and communication, and in order to provide a focus for treatment. Broadly speaking, I think that many patients can be classified in clinical practice using the organic categories of delirium (for symptoms of acute schizophrenia), dementia (chronic, negative-state schizophrenia), and the secondary drug side-effects of treating primary symptoms.

The extent to which negative symptoms may be a consequence of neuroleptic treatment of positive symptoms was pointed out by David Healy, who has also published a fascinating study of the effects of the neuroleptic droperidol in normal volunteers (Healy and Farquhar, 1998). Some of the chronic psychotic patients who currently attract a diagnosis of schizophrenia may of course also suffer from other symptoms such as malaise, anxiety, fatigue, etc., and these may have further treatment implications.

It is important to get away from the automatic equation of a schizophrenic diagnosis with neuroleptic ('antipsychotic') drug treatment, as if schizophrenia was a disease and neuroleptics had some kind of fundamental anti-disease activity. This is based on the seriously mistaken assumption that neuroleptics correct a brain abnormality in schizophrenia in the same kind of way as L-dopa (partly) corrects a brain abnormality in Parkinson's disease. Instead, treatment should be symptomatic and aimed primarily at making patients *feel better*. Treatment should therefore be tailored to individual patients on the basis of focusing on their dominant symptoms using the safest drugs with the least debilitating side-effects, and involving (ideally) a therapeutic partnership with the patient and (at least) serious attempts to understand the patient's subjective response to treatment. This strategy, which is superbly expounded in Healy's *Psychiatric Drugs Explained*, needs to be evaluated against current practice.

References

Healy D (1997) *Psychiatric Drugs Explained*. London: Mosby.

Healy D and Farquhar G (1998) Immediate effects of droperidol. *Hum Psychopharmacol Clin Exp.* **13**: 113–20.

Chapter 13 – Psychopharmacology and the human condition

In addition to the references below, the work of David Pearce has been of substantial help in clarifying the issues in relation to human happiness. Dave hosts an astonishing group of websites, which can be accessed via www. neuropharmacology.com

Further reading

Barkow JH (1992) Beneath new culture is old psychology: gossip and social stratification. In: JH Barkow, L Cosmides and J Tooby (eds) *The Adapted Mind*. New York: Oxford University Press, 627–37.

Barkow JH, Cosmides L and Tooby J (eds) (1992) *The Adapted Mind*. New York: Oxford University Press.

Charlton BG (1997) A syllabus for evolutionary medicine. *J R Soc Med*. **90**: 397–9.

Charlton BG (1998) Psychopharmacology and the human condition. *J R Soc Med*. **91**: 599–601.

Damasio, AR (1994) *Descartes' Error: Emotion, Reason and the Human Brain*. New York: Putnam.

Dunbar R (1995) *Grooming, Gossip and the Evolution of Language*. London: Faber.

Healy D (1998) *The Antidepressant Era*. Cambridge, MA: Harvard University Press.

Kramer PD (1994) *Listening to Prozac*. London: Fourth Estate.

Knutson B, Wolkowitz OM, Cole SW, Chan T, Moore EA, Johnson RC, Terpestra J, Turner RA and Reus VI (1998) Selective alteration of personality and social behavior by serotonergic intervention. *Am J Psychiatry*. **155**: 373–9.

Nesse RM (1997) Psychoactive drug use in evolutionary perspective. *Science*. **278**: 63–6.

Verkes RJ, Van der Mast RC, Hengeveld MW, Twyl JP, Zwinderman AH and Van Kempen EM (1998) Reduction by paroxetine of suicidal behavior in patients with repeated suicide attempts but not major depression. *Am J Psychiatry*. **155**: 543–7.

APPENDIX 1 – Evolution and the cognitive neuroscience of awareness, consciousness and language

This section is just plain difficult! I have done my best to make things clear, particularly by the use of examples, but I found this very hard to grasp (I read Damasio's book four times before I really understood it), and it is likely that you will find it difficult, too. However, it is just about as important as science gets...

Evolution of awareness

My understanding of the nature and role of awareness depends upon Francis Crick's *The Astonishing Hypotheses*, although what Crick terms 'consciousness' I would term 'awareness'. I found Zeki's *A Vision of the Brain* extremely useful for understanding the general organisation of the brain as revealed by vision researchers. I have also drawn heavily upon the work and conversation of my colleagues at the Psychology Department of Newcastle University who are active in visual research and cortical connectivity, especially Malcolm Young, Jack Scannell, Martin Tovee and Piers Cornelissen.

Evolution of consciousness

The key to understanding the nature of consciousness is the somatic marker mechanism as described by Antonio Damasio in *Descartes' Error*. However, while Damasio describes many of the things that consciousness *does* and what happens when consciousness is absent (in patients with brain damage), he does not say why consciousness *evolved*. This is my concern here – to describe the nature of the social selection pressure for evolving consciousness, and the specific nature of the social task performed by this general mechanism. Thus the neural nature of the somatic marker mechanism needs to be combined with an understanding of the nature of strategic social intelligence.

The somatic marker mechanism

I would consider Damasio's concept of the somatic marker mechanism to be one of the most fruitful ideas I have encountered. However, it is a difficult concept to grasp on paper (although it is easier to explain verbally), which may account for its otherwise astonishing lack of major impact to date. One difficulty is that the somatic marker mechanism overlaps conceptually with 'consciousness' and 'theory of mind', which are also slippery and elusive ideas. I have striven to bring some terminological clarity and precision to these matters, since the concepts themselves are not so difficult as the terminological tangle can make them appear. I have equated the somatic marker mechanism with consciousness, suggested that the function of consciousness is strategic social intelligence, and proposed that theory of mind is based upon the somatic marker mechanism, but with the addition of abstract symbolic language in humans, which introduces a new set of possibilities for what is represented.

Language

Language is another terminological and conceptual minefield. This chapter was immeasurably helped by discussions with Tina Fry over a period of about two years. Tina is trained in linguistics, and we are working together on the evolution of language. Most of the new ideas relating to the concept of displacement – the crucial aspect of displacement, the mechanism of displacement by association in working memory, the putative ecological conditions for language evolution, and so on – were developed in the course of discussions with Tina, and as a consequence of her knowledge. She has taught me a tremendous amount, and has by and large eliminated some of my grossest errors, but there are a few issues over which I have defied her advice, and for which I take full responsibility.

Further reading

Adolphs R, Damasio H, Tranel D and Damasio AR (1996) Cortical systems for the recognition of emotion in facial expressions. *J Neurosci.* **16**: 7678–87.

Baron-Cohen S (1990) Autism: a specific cognitive disorder of 'mind-blindness'. *Int Rev Psychiatry.* **2**: 81–90.

Baron-Cohen S (1995) *Mind-Blindness: an Essay on Autism and Theory of Mind.* Cambridge, MA: MIT Press.

Barton RA and Dunbar RIM (1997) Evolution of the social brain. In: A Whiten and RW Byrne (eds) *Machiavellian Intelligence II: Extensions and Evaluations.* Cambridge: Cambridge University Press, 240–63.

Bechara A, Damasio AR, Damasio H and Anderson SW (1994) Insensitivity to future consequence following damage to human prefrontal cortex. *Cognition.* **50**: 7–15.

Bechara A, Tranel D, Damasio H and Damasio AR (1996) Failure to respond automatically to anticipated future outcomes following damage to prefrontal cortex. *Cereb Cortex.* **6**: 215–25.

Bechara A, Damasio H, Tranel D and Damasio AR (1997) Deciding advantageously before knowing the advantageous strategy. *Science.* **275**: 1293–5.

Bradshaw JL (1997) *Human Evolution: a Neuropsychological Perspective.* London: Psychology Press.

Byrne RW (1995) *The Thinking Ape: Evolutionary Origins of Intelligence.* Oxford: Oxford University Press.

Byrne RW and Whiten A (eds) (1988) *Machiavellian Intelligence: Social Expertise and the Evolution of Intellect in Monkeys, Apes and Humans.* Oxford: Clarendon Press.

Carruthers P and Smith PK (eds) (1996) *Theories of Mind.* Cambridge: Cambridge University Press.

Charlton BG (1995) Cognitive neuropsychiatry and the future of diagnosis: a 'PC' model of the mind. *Br J Psychiatry.* **167**: 149–53.

Charlton BG (1997) The inequity of inequality: egalitarian instincts and evolutionary psychology. *J Health Psychol.* **2**: 413–25.

Crick F (1994) *The Astonishing Hypothesis: the Scientific Search for the Soul.* London: Touchstone.

Crick FC and Jones E (1993) Backwardness of human neuroanatomy. *Nature.* **361**: 109–10.

Crick F and Koch C (1995) Are we aware of neural activity in primary visual cortex? *Nature.* **375**: 121–3.

Damasio AR (1994) *Descartes' Error: Emotion, Reason and the Human Brain.* London: Macmillan.

Damasio AR (1995) Towards a neurobiology of emotion and feeling: operational concepts and hypotheses. *Neuroscientist.* **1**: 19–25.

Damasio AR (1996) The somatic marker hypothesis and the possible functions of the prefrontal cortex. *Philos Trans R Soc Lond.* **351**: 1413–20.

Damasio AR and Damasio H (1994) Cortical systems for retrieval of concrete knowledge: the convergence zone framework. In: C Koch (ed.) *Large-Scale Neuronal Theories of the Brain.* Cambridge, MA: MIT Press, 61–74.

Dunbar R (1996) *Grooming, Gossip and the Evolution of Language.* London: Faber.

Foley R (1993) Causes and consequences in human evolution. *J R Anthropol Inst.* **1**: 67–86.

Foley R (1995) *Humans Before Humanity.* Oxford: Basil Blackwell.

Gazzaniga MR (ed.) (1995) *The Cognitive Neurosciences.* Cambridge, MA: MIT Press.

Goldman-Rakic PS (1995) Cellular basis of working memory. *Neuron.* **14**: 477–85.

Humphrey NK (1976) The social function of intellect. In: PPG Bateson and RA Hinde (eds) *Growing Points in Ethology.* Cambridge: Cambridge University Press.

Kummer H (1995) *In Quest of the Sacred Baboon: a Scientist's Journey.* New Jersey: Princeton University Press.

Mithen S (1996) *The Prehistory of Mind.* London: Thames and Hudson.

Pinker S (1994) *The Language Instinct.* New York: William Morrow.

Savage-Rumbaugh S, Shanker S and Taylor TJ (1998) *Apes, Language and the Human Mind.* New York: Oxford University Press.

Seyfarth RM and Cheney DL (1994) The evolution of social cognition in primates. In: LA Real (ed.) *Behavioural Mechanisms in Evolutionary Ecology*. Chicago: University of Chicago Press, 371–89.

Shallice T (1988) *From Neuropsychology to Mental Structure*. Cambridge: Cambridge University Press.

Tovee MJ (1994) Neuronal processing: how fast is the speed of thought? *Curr Biol.* **4**: 1125–7.

Whiten A and Byrne RW (eds) (1997) *Machiavellian Intelligence II: Extensions and Evaluations*. Cambridge: Cambridge University Press.

Wierzbicka A (1994) Cognitive domains and the structure of the lexicon: the case of the emotions. In: LA Hirschfield and SA Gelman (eds) *Mapping the Mind: Domain Specificity in Cognition and Culture*. Cambridge: Cambridge University Press, 431–52.

Worden R (1995) A speed limit for evolution. *J Theor Biol.* **176**: 137–52.

Young MP (1992) Objective analysis of the topological organization of the primate cortical visual system. *Nature.* **358**: 152–4.

Young MP, Scannell JW, O'Neill MA, Hilgetag CC, Burns G and Blakemore C (1995) Non-metric multi-dimensional scaling in the analysis of neuroanatomical connection data and the organization of the primate cortical visual system. *Phil Trans R Soc Lond.* **348**: 281–308.

Zeki S (1993) *A Vision of the Brain*. Oxford: Blackwell Scientific Publications.

Appendix 2 – Human creativity and the *Col-oh-nell Flastratus* phenomenon

I have enjoyed the work of Abraham Maslow ever since I was introduced to it by Colin Wilson's book, *New Pathways in Psychology: Maslow and the Post-Freudian Revolution*. The moments of subjective delight and insight described as 'peak experiences' *feel* important, and they deserve exploration. The form of the peak experience seems biologically explicable in terms of the somatic marker mechanism, and the fact that we impose story-like explanations appears to be an aspect of human social intelligence, but the *content* of the experience is individually and culturally variable – and the validity of even the most subjectively compelling content is fascinatingly uncertain.

Further reading

Bronowski J (1975) *Science and Human Values* (revised edition). New York: Harper & Row.

Bronowski J (1977) *A Sense of the Future.* Cambridge, MA: MIT Press.

Cairns Smith AG (1996) *Evolving the Mind: on the Nature of Matter and the Origin of Consciousness.* Cambridge: Cambridge University Press.

Crick F (1990) *What Mad Pursuit: a Personal View of Scientific Discovery.* Harmondsworth: Penguin.

Crick F (1994) *The Astonishing Hypothesis: the Scientific Search for the Soul.* London: Touchstone.

Freeland Judson H (1995) *The Eighth Day of Creation: Makers of the Revolution in Biology.* Harmondsworth: Penguin.

Gleik J (1992) *Genius: Richard Feynman and Modern Physics.* London: Little, Brown & Co.

Graves R (1948) *The White Goddess: a Historical Grammar of Poetic Myth.* London: Faber and Faber.

'Horizon' – BBC Television (1996) *Fermat's Last Theorem* – (transcript). London: British Broadcasting Corporation.

Hull D (1988) *Science as a Process.* Chicago: University of Chicago Press.

Huxley A (1959) *The Doors of Experience.* Harmondsworth: Penguin (first published in 1954).

James W (1982) *The Varieties of Religious Experience.* Harmondsworth: Penguin (reissue, first published in 1902).

Maslow A (1983) *Motivation and Personality* (3e). New York: Harper and Row.

Szilard L (1978) *Leo Szilard: his Version of the Facts.* Cambridge, MA: MIT Press.

White M and Gribbin J (1993) *Einstein: a Life in Science.* London: Simon and Schuster.

Wilson C (1972) *New Pathways in Psychology: Maslow and the Post-Freudian Revolution.* London: Gollancz.

Ziman J (1978) *Reliable Knowledge: an Exploration of the Grounds for Belief in Science.* New York: Cambridge University Press.

Index